EATING FOR ENERGY

Transforming Your Life Through Living

Plant-Based Whole Foods.

Disclaimer

The information and recommendations in this book are for information purposes only. None of the information herein should be construed as a claim for cure, treatment or prevention of disease. All matters regarding physical health should be referred to a qualified health-care professional. Consult a health-care professional before beginning any fitness or nutrition program. Total Wellness Consulting does not claim any responsibility for the misuse of the information within this book.

Claim Your **<u>FREE</u>** *Eating for Energy*

Book Bonuses Today!

Go to...

www.totalwellnessconsulting.ca/book_bonuses.html

...and get tons of great bonuses that will complement

what you're about to read!

Help Us Help Others

Please help us spread the word of living nutrition, optimal health, and vitality...
Tell at least 3 friends about this book.

10% of all profits from this book go to charities (such as the *Fruit Tree Planting Foundation* and *United Way*) that promote sustainable agriculture and the health of our planet and its communities. Thank you for your support!

A Few Testimonials to Wet Your Appetite
(No pun intended!)

"In a world filled with dubious diet books, Eating for Energy identifies the proven steps that will lead to abundant health, a fit body, and radiant energy. I can't think of a better book on healthy eating to help you get from where you are to where you want to be. It is easy, understandable, inspiring, and applicable. It's the best tool to come along in years."

Raymond Aaron
New York Times Top Ten Best Selling Author
Chicken Soup for the Parent's Soul

"I found Yuri Elkaim's book Eating For Energy surprisingly innovative. The entire book is framed positively and contains a wealth of solution-oriented action steps for readers. The recipes are quite extensive as well. Enjoy Eating For Energy and Have The Best Day Ever!"

David Wolfe
Founder of www.sunfood.com, www.ftpf.org, thebestdayever.com, and author of The *Sunfood Diet Success System*, *Naked Chocolate*, *Amazing Grace*, and *Eating For Beauty*.

"Medicine today should encompass a multidisciplinary approach to health promotion and health prevention. Yuri Elkaim's Eating for Energy tackles heath promotion from the most basic building blocks of life, namely, diet. Healthy dietary lifestyle choices serve to increase one's energy, productivity and prevent disease. Yuri's e-book sheds light on dietary choices in a comprehensive, yet simplistic approach. Everyone can benefit from his knowledge and insight into healthy eating. I highly recommend reading this book."

Dr. Danny Grossi, BSc., MSc., MD
Clinic Director
Toronto Regional Pain Management Centre

"I'm sure you've heard the idea at some point that you never know how unhealthy you were until you become really healthy. I have always considered myself 'healthy'; eating what I thought was right, exercising and enjoying a balanced lifestyle. What Yuri's book, Eating for Energy helped me to understand is by making some simple adjustments to my current lifestyle and eating habits, I could feel Great! After reading his book I have more much energy and I look and feel lighter. Thanks Yuri!"

TL Bonnar
General Manager
Avalon Woods – Health Club for Mature Adults

"In this book, "Eating for Energy", Yuri has a natural way of explaining nutritional concepts in a way that makes them easy to grasp. His enthusiasm and passion for nutrition is matched only by his passion for fitness, and it truly shows through his writing style - this makes "Eating for Energy" not only educational, but also a fun and exciting read!

As a naturopathic doctor, I see a wide range of health concerns in my practice ranging from severe skin conditions to digestive disorders to chronic inflammatory diseases that are aggravated or even caused by unhealthy eating. The "Eating for Energy" 12-Week Meal Plan and huge compendium of healthy and tasty recipes provides a complete and effective program to transition people to a lifestyle of healthy eating that will lead to many positive health ramifications.

I highly recommend "Eating for Energy" to anyone who is interested in bettering their health through diet and has not found a resource that provides them with the motivation and education to do so."

Makoto Trotter, B.Sc., N.D.
Naturopathic Doctor
Clinic Director
Zen-tai Wellness Centre

"I am still in the process of reading your book, "Eating for Energy", and wanted to let you know how blown away I am! I've searched the world (World Wide Web, anyway) over, searching for an understandable, do-able nutrition plan that would support my athletic lifestyle, my post-menopausal condition, AND give me the best health of my life...and I've found it! I also appreciate your forum and the personalized tips you shared with me. You're the nutritional/fitness guru I've been searching for, and I'm forever grateful"!

Kathy Roberts

"I've been living a vegan lifestyle for the past 2 years, but "Eating for Energy" has catapulted my commitment to nutrition, my health, and my energy to an entirely new, amazing, & exciting level! It is the most down-to-earth, concise, and simple approach to living a life of vibrancy. I have never felt better in my life!!!! And the simple recipes included are DELICIOUS. The entire world should read Yuri's book"!

Amy Miller

"I am almost half way through the Eating for Energy and it has given me a great foundation on energy and nutrition. I now know which foods will contribute to better health and why. A good example is the fact you can get your daily calcium out of 100 grams of sesame seeds compared to 5 glasses of milk! I can't wait to finish the rest of the book. "

Colin Nanka
Toronto, Canada

This book is dedicated to **YOU**

May you enjoy the health and happiness that you deserve!

'The future is not a result of choices among alternative paths offered by the present, but a place that is created - created first in the mind and will, created next in activity. The future is not some place we are going to, but one we are creating. The paths are not to be found, but made, and the activity of making them, changes both the maker and the destination."

- Deborah James
Business Consultant

Remember to log on to our **Fit Forum** to get all your questions answered, share your experiences with other users, and to post any new living food recipes that you might have. Just click on the Eating for Energy forum and post away!

Visit **www.totalwellnessconsulting.ca/book_bonuses.html**

Sincerely,

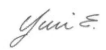

Table of Contents

Eating for Energy

Understanding the Nutritional Lifestyle

Eating for Energy

Living the Nutritional Lifestyle Success Guide

EATING FOR ENERGY

Understanding the Nutritional Lifestyle

1 My Reason Why

Welcome to a new world of possibilities.

I cannot express how excited am I to share with you the wonderful information contained within the *Eating for Energy* program! As you read through these pages, my hope is that you discover the tremendous importance of this philosophy not only for your own health and performance but for the health of the world as a whole. This book will show you the importance and need for eating living plant-based whole foods for the best possible health, energy, performance, and body that you deserve. No other time in history has this information been as needed as it is now. If you apply even just 10% of the teachings in this book your life will transform dramatically!

I decided that I needed to write *Eating for Energy* because of the ailing state of our world and the people within it. Without a doubt the 21st century is the greatest time in history to be alive, yet billions of people are suffering. Our planet is suffering. People from all walks of life are no healthier today than were the ancient civilizations from thousands of years prior. In fact, they're less healthy! Sure we're living longer but are we living in the best health possible? Definitely not!

The motivation for this book stems from several personal, family, client, and society-wide experiences.

Our Current "ill – State" of Affairs

It's not rocket science that the state of health in the western world is far from optimal. Heart disease, cancer, and diabetes – the most common diseases in the western world – are truly out of control. These diseases are those of the least concern in Latin American, African, and even Asian countries. They obviously have their diseases to contend with but they are to a lesser extent influenced by lifestyle as are the "Big 3" illnesses of western countries. Just think of the amount of people that you know who suffer from either one or all of these diseases. It's absolutely staggering!

According to the **American Cancer Society**, men have a 1 in 2 chance of developing cancer in their lifetime; while for women, the risk is a little more than 1 in 3, with 77% of all cases occurring in people who are older than 55 years of age.[1] However, I personally know several men in their early 30's who have been diagnosed with prostate cancer! Fortunately, they have all overcome the disease. Only about 5% of all cancers are strongly hereditary with the remaining 95% of cases being a result of damage (mutation) to genes that occur during one's lifetime.[2] These mutations (mainly caused by free radical damage) may occur from a variety of exogenous sources including tobacco, excessive sunlight, x-rays, chemicals (including those in foods), and more. Lung and bronchial cancer are still the most prevalent forms of cancer among both men and women, and the numbers are rising. The incidence of breast, colorectal, and prostate cancers are all starting to decline.

On a positive note, the 5-year relative survival rate for all diagnosed cancers between 1996 and 2002 is 66%, up from 51% in 1975-1977. The improvement in survival reflects advancements in early detection and improvements in treatment. As with most lifestyle-related diseases, cancer is more easily prevented than treated, hence the importance of proper nutrition and a healthy lifestyle.

---

[1] American Cancer Society. *Cancer Facts and Figures 2007*. Atlanta: American Cancer Society 2007.

[2] American Cancer Society. *Cancer Facts and Figures 2007*. Atlanta: American Cancer Society 2007.

Fatter Than Ever Before!

Being overweight is a major risk factor for all disease. Unfortunately, we are dealing with an epidemic of obesity as people are inundated with poor food choices, chemically induced addictive foods, and a lack physical activity, especially in North America. According to **Statistics Canada (2004)**, 59.2% of Canadians are overweight or obese (36% are overweight, 23% are obese)![3] Similar numbers (actually slightly higher) are seen in the United States.

The risk of being overweight is highly correlated with diet and lifestyle. According to another report by **Statistics Canada in 2006**, children and youth who ate fruits and vegetables at least 5 times a day were substantially less likely to be overweight than their counterparts who did not. Furthermore, the likelihood of being overweight/obese rose as "screen time" (watching TV, playing video games) increased.[4]

Whatever happened to playing outside or taking a walk instead of flopping down on the couch for several hours to watch the latest reality TV shows? When I was young I don't even remember going to school! My childhood was filled with road hockey, soccer, and playing adventure games outside – I even suffered from bad asthma which forced me to take breaks every 10 minutes. But that didn't deter me! To this day, I have ensured that play and activity remain a priority in my life. I can't even imagine what my life would be like otherwise. Applying the same (or even greater) importance on quality nutrition is absolutely paramount. I truly believe that we can prevent and/or deal with 95% of all sickness and diseases through excellent nutrition, regular exercise, and stress management.

Eating for Energy will educate you and then hold your hand, serving as your guide as you transition into making healthier food choices for the best and healthiest life ever!

---

[3] Statistics Canada (2004). *Canadian Community Health Survey: Nutrition.* Statistics Canada.

[4] Statistics Canada Health Report, vol. 17, no. 3, August 2006.

To further illustrate the importance of this book allow me to present some more startling nutritional findings. Consider the findings from a recent survey entitled **"The Changing Canadian Diet – A Report Card"** by Canada Food Stats. Although Canadian-based, many of these trends are reflective of all North American habits. Between 1970 and 2004, the consumption of fats & oils increased from 15 to 25 kg/person/year. The consumption of wheat flour increased from 45 to 53 kg/person/year. The intake of cheeses – from 4 to 9 kg/person/year.[5]

However, there are some positive trends as well. During the same time frame, the consumption of vegetables and fruits saw a steady increase; while a decline in beef and milk was also apparent.

Things are starting to improve, but we have a long way to go. My mission is to inspire you to realize that settling for mediocre health and energy is not acceptable! You deserve to feel radiant energy each and every day. You were put on this planet to achieve your full potential. You were born to be the best you can be at what you do. Food is one of the most powerful tools available to help you reach your true potential! By following the principles outlined in this book you will see what I mean. Whether it be to gain more energy, lose weight, perform better in your sport, or simply to prevent disease – it can and will be yours!

My Own Experience

As a former professional soccer player I can personally attest to what proper nutrition has meant in my life. In my playing days, after having graduated as a Kinesiologist, I thought I had a pretty good handle on what healthy eating was all about. In fact, when I played in France, my French teammates used to call me "Mr. Vitamine" – the translation is pretty obvious.

---

[5] Canada Food Stats, November 2005.

A typical day for me would begin with Corn Flakes topped with chopped up banana, strawberries, kiwi, and 2% milk. Hmmm... sounds pretty good doesn't it?! About 2 hrs later I would be off to our morning training session. After having exhausted myself during practice, I would come back home for lunch and prepare myself a beautiful pasta with all kinds of vegetables and some diced chicken breast or canned tuna.

However, I never stopped to think about why I constantly needed to take a nap during the afternoon. Was I over-trained? Was I not sleeping well? The signs led me to believe that everything was in check. Yet, there was something that just wasn't right. My energy was low (compared to now) and my performance was beginning to suffer. Nonetheless, I was having a great time pursuing my life's passion (at least formerly) and was determined to put my troubles aside.

Having worked with hundreds of elite level athletes I now know that my experience was not unique.

Several years after ending my soccer career, I decided to pursue studies in nutrition. I had always been interested in understanding why we all respond differently to the same foods. I wanted to see if what I was doing was working, and obviously it wasn't! I always felt that nutritional science was a vast and undiscovered universe. I desperately wanted to learn more so I could better help myself and others.

So, I embarked upon studies in Holistic Nutrition, and gratefully so. This intense 1 year program at the Canadian School of Natural Nutrition opened my eyes to a completely different way of viewing food, the human body, and the interaction of both. The knowledge I acquired was far beyond what I could have ever imagined and I feel compelled to share it with the world.

During my studies I began uncovering reasons and solutions to a condition I had developed when I was 17 years old, called Alopecia. This is an auto-immune condition whereby the body attacks its hair follicles. In my senior year of high school I had lost all of my hair. I went to allergists, dermatologists, and every specialist in between. The only so-called "solution" was to get cortisone injections, and that *really* irritated me. I wanted to get to the root of the problem, and not just cover up the symptoms with prescription drugs.

As I dove into studying nutrition and its impact on the body I began to discover that my condition, which apparently had no known cause or solution, could in fact be "heavily" related to the foods I was eating and the health and integrity of my digestive tract! This blew my mind and to this day I am making the necessary progress nutritionally to overcome Alopecia, although I'm quite happy with my easy-to-maintain shaved head. These are nutritional principles you'll learn about in this book and that will tremendously benefit you no matter your situation.

After all, Hippocrates once said…

> *"Let food be your medicine, and medicine your food"*

The Story of Bestafar

I always tell the story of my late Bestafar (Danish, for grandfather) who was in great health until his early 70's. He lived in Adelaide, Australia where he gardened each day, spent a great deal of time walking, eating relatively healthy foods, and spending quality time with family. Then, decades later he decided to move back to Oshawa, Ontario (in Canada) where he returned to live in the same "gloomy" apartment he had left roughly 20 years prior. He was about 75 years old at this point.

As a young admirer of my grandfather I was always amazed at how fast and sharp he was when playing cards, talking about current events, and even when watching the Price is Right (I think he watched this more so for the lovely ladies). But as the years passed he began to slow down and his health deteriorated noticeably. He had not maintained his healthy Australian lifestyle and became much more sedentary while losing the motivation to prepare healthy meals for himself. Within a short period of time he had to have his gall bladder removed, was diagnosed with prostate cancer, and eventually developed Parkinson's-like symptoms. He was 91 when he passed away in late 2006.

In his later years it always upset me to hear responses like *"There's no use complaining"* or *"Not that great"* when I asked him how he was doing. We speak our lives. You can tell a whole lot about someone by the dialogue they employ. My grandfather was not using a dialogue that demonstrated vibrant health or even an optimistic outlook.

My grandfather's experience is just one of the reasons I wrote *Eating for Energy*. I am extremely passionate about helping people live their best possible lives and it frustrates me to no end when, for whatever reason, they don't. Unfortunately, as human beings we are retroactive in nature, meaning that we don't act until after the fact. I have always promoted a proactive approach to healthy living. It is my personal mission to inspire and motivate as many people as I can to do the same – including you!

I want you to realize right now that who you are is not necessarily who you *really* are. What I mean is that **you are not what you are, rather, what you are, is what you can be**. In essence, you are your potential! You have incredible potential! You have unbelievable potential, and I know that you know it! You have a feeling deep down inside of you that is burning to express itself. That flickering flame may represent your desire to achieve unbelievable health and radiance or maybe even to pursue a vocation that you absolutely love. The key is to remember that your potential is endless. You can achieve whatever you want.

Stories from My Personal Clients

(The names have been changed to protect the innocent)

The following are several real life examples from some of my personal fitness clients. They are all active individuals with goals of attaining greater physical and mental well-being. You can see for yourself that some major nutritional work was recommended.

Julie, a tax specialist with a big accounting firm, was regularly drinking 3-4 cups of coffee per day, had mid-afternoon sugar cravings which would normally be satisfied by pastries, chocolate, etc... and rarely drank water.

Debra, a young and trendy advertising creative director, was so concerned with losing 10 pounds but her daily food intake consisted of a morning pastry, take-out for lunch, and popcorn and candy for dinner (and that was a good day). She wanted a magic "supplement" that would compensate for her diet and was unwilling to adjust any of her dietary choices.

Melissa, a retired business owner, would complain of frequent heart burn symptoms (which was actually a hiatal hernia) and digestive difficulty, yet was reluctant to reduce her consumption of heavy animal protein and starchy meals.

Rose, a mental health nurse, was one of my first clients and also became a good friend. She would regularly consume 6-10 diet sodas per day!

These 4 clients have been highlighted for no other reason than to illustrate that even health/fitness-conscious people don't necessarily know and/or employ the principles of healthy eating. It is very important to remember that **you can be fit without being healthy!** Obviously, after applying several of the principles you will learn in this book, these wonderful clients have made tremendous improvements in their dietary habits.

I have always been fit but not necessarily healthy. Not until I restructured the way I ate did things start to fall into place. Aside from a bout of food poisoning from some suspect Indian food a few years ago, I can't remember the last time I was sick.

Several of the clients mentioned above would call me to cancel an exercise session due to the flu, bad allergies, the common cold, headaches, and many other reasons. I couldn't believe how often the same people could get sick in a single year! If I remember correctly, I had one client who was sick on about 8 different occasions in just 1 year!

You are what you eat. You are also what your foods eat. You need to strongly re-evaluate the foods that you put into your mouth. I've always told my clients that nutrition accounts for 80% of the battle. Whether you're looking for increased energy, weight loss, better health, or greater performance it all comes down to what foods you are eating and how well your body processes them.

You need to see yourself as a Ferrari. Would you put anything but the best fuel into your Ferrari? Obviously not! And if you said yes, then I'd be happy to take that poor car off your hands. So, if you would fuel your Ferrari with the best, then why wouldn't you do the same for yourself? In fact, you are much greater than a Ferrari! You deserve only the best possible foods to fuel your body. You must not settle for anything less or your "engine" will wear down and your performance will suffer.

I strongly believe we can prevent and solve all disease known to mankind. I've seen it with my own two eyes. I've seen people with Multiple Sclerosis dramatically regain their quality of life through proper nutrition. I've seen obese people return to and maintain their intended weight through proper eating and active living. I've seen hypertension and other cardiovascular complications reversed through proper nutrition. I've seen athletic performance go from dismally lethargic to unbounded endurance, strength, and power - All through the principles outlined in this book!

As you will learn, the principles in *Eating for Energy* apply across the board and will have a dramatic and profound benefit on your health and quality of life. These are principles that have been around for millions of years yet have been suppressed by technological innovation, big business, government recommendations, and a lack of understanding of the interaction between foods and the human body.

Think about where we came from and what nature intended for us to thrive. That's where we're going!

An Old New Way of Viewing Foods

If you're reading this book, then you're probably searching for something that you currently are not experiencing. Perhaps you want to feel more energetic, improve your health status, recover from disease, get rid of allergies, dramatically improve your physical performance, or even lose weight. Whatever your reason, I feel privileged to help you attain your objectives and I thank you for allowing me to guide you through your transformation.

What you'll find in these pages is a new way of looking at food. I have no interest in presenting a typical "medical" approach to "supposed" healthy eating. My intention is to empower you with amazing insight into how your body operates at the cellular level and how every single food you put in your mouth either enlivens or drains you!

You will learn some principles which may seem absolutely unconventional to what you've been told. And that's great! As a former professional soccer player who thought he had a clean diet, I was astonished when I began to experience the teachings of *Eating for Energy*. I have always been a fairly knowledgeable person, yet always willing to learn. As mentioned earlier, I used to believe that eating a large serving of cooked pasta a few hours before training or a game was what I was supposed to do. I even remember waking up in the morning each day to Corn Flakes topped with banana, kiwi, strawberries and smothered in 2% cow's milk. *"WOW, I'm eating so amazingly healthy"* is what I used to believe. But when I look back onto my playing days and recount the fatigue and digestive issues I experienced, I almost wish I could go back and do it all again with my new approach.

The information in this book comes from my years of study and practical experience in health and wellness that ultimately led me into the field of holistic nutrition. What intrigues me most about nutrition is the myriad of ways the body can react to food. We are all unique in our biochemical makeup, yet we are all human, and have roughly 99.993% similar DNA. This means there is an approach to nutrition that can apply to and dramatically help at least 98% of the population. That approach is what you'll be introduced to in this book.

Once you understand how your body works and how it is connected to the foods you eat, you will begin to realize what I mean.

At the end of each chapter in the first part of this book, I've included action steps for you to take. Knowledge is power, but only if it is applied. Reading the contents of this book is great but you need to actually apply its teachings to reap the benefits. Action, action, action! That's what it's all about. We all know everything don't we? We know that it's important to exercise and which foods to avoid but how many of us actually follow through and do what we know? Not many.

So use this book as your guide. Make notes, benefit from its information and do your best to take the action steps and recommendations outlined.

1 Action Steps

My Reason Why

1. Begin a journal to track your progress as you move through this program. Note how you feel throughout your day. When do you get hungry? When do you eat, and what do you eat? What emotions do you experience before, during, and after you eat? Write down whatever you can to give yourself greater insight as you move forward in your journey. You can download your FREE food journal when you visit **www.totalwellnessconsulting.ca/book_bonuses.html**.

2. Before beginning the program take a "before" photo and any appropriate measurements and/or indicators if you wish. This will give you another means of comparison as you move through *Eating for Energy*. It's easy to forget just how far you've come, so this gentle reminder may give you powerful leverage to reach your goals.

3. Write down 3 important goals that you **need** to achieve and why you need to achieve them. Have the goals visible and read them aloud at least once per day. I would recommend you write them down as if they've already been attained.

   Here's an example:

   "I am so happy and grateful now that...."

2 Planting the Seeds of Foundation

We are all connected. Human beings, animals, plants, all species, and our beautiful planet are parts of a whole. But, in order to help our planet, we must first help ourselves.

Our "ill" planet is nothing more than a mirror image of what is happening within each one of us and society as a whole. Therefore, you must first spend time on developing and "cleansing" yourself before anything in your outer world will change.

When you strive to become better yourself, everything around you will become better as well. The environment in which you live, the people that surround you and all of life's situations will improve as you do. By working on yourself, focusing on maintaining a healthy, positive outlook, and being happy you can begin to experience health, joy, and energy in endless abundance.

In order for this to occur you must begin to take 100% responsibility for your actions. It is important to remember that each action yields a result: cause and effect. Take full responsibility for everything that happens in your life – good or bad. Winners take full responsibility for everything that happens to them. They acknowledge when they do things well and admit when they're at fault.

The focus of *Eating for Energy* is on vibrant, superior, and energetic health! If you are suffering from ill health, there is only one person responsible – yourself. Blaming others or circumstances will not empower you. To achieve ultimate health, you must take 100% responsibility.

The question I pose to you is this:

"How badly do you want to look and feel amazing, have abundant energy, live in radiant health, eliminate fatigue, lose weight, improve your performance, and live a long and youthful life?"

When the emotional desire for a thing is so intense that it illuminates every fiber of your being, it shall then be fulfilled – and not a moment sooner. What you focus on expands. Focus on what you want and it will come into your life. Whether it be an ideal body weight, greater energy, youthfulness, or anything else – simply focus your thoughts and emotions on your desires and they shall be yours.

Like attracts like and things produce after their own kind. Banana trees will yield bananas and orange trees will yield oranges. Once seeds are planted they sprout and grow into physical realities. And just as orange seeds will not grow into banana tress, nor will negative thoughts grow into positive physical realities.

Your mind is without a doubt the most fertile soil in the world. For what you sow, you shall reap. If you plant seeds of despair, anger, frustration, and stress you shall grow weeds (or physical realities) that reflect these same things. On the other hand, if you plant seeds of love, happiness, optimism, and radiant health, you shall grow glorious trees of abundance in your life.

For many people, thinking in the positive on a consistent basis is challenging. We have a tendency to complain. Have you ever noticed how people try to out-complain each other? You tell a friend that something bad happened to you over the weekend only to hear them respond with something even more tragic that happened to them. It becomes a battle of who's got the worst life! You must eliminate this tendency, or the precise things you complain about will continually resurface in your life.

It's time to live a life of endless abundance – a life full of radiant energy and optimal health.

By following the aforementioned guidelines as well as the nutrition concepts in this book you will notice the following:

- Greater productivity at work or in your business
- Greater athletic performance and quicker recovery
- Healthy, long-term and sustained weight loss (if desired)
- Healthier skin, hair, and nails – you will have a glow!
- Dramatically improved energy and vigor
- More motivation
- Less fear and more willingness to take challenges head-on
- Ability to prevent sickness and disease
- Increased chance of prolonging your life while living in great health (my current goal is to live to 200 years of age!)

- And much more…

2 Action Steps

Planting the Seeds of Foundation

1. Spend at least 5 minutes each morning expressing sincere gratitude for everything you have in your life. Until you're grateful for what you have, you won't get any more. This is also a terrific way to minimize stress in your life.

2. I challenge you to not complain for a full 7 days! It's not as easy as it sounds. Each time you catch yourself complaining in anyway shape or form you must start again at day 0. I know you can do it.

3. With absolute conviction affirm the following to yourself each day:

   "I am responsible for my glowing health. I create my health and deserve every ounce of it!"

   "I am whole, perfect, energetic, joyful, harmonious, and loving"

   Special Bonus: Go to **www.totalwellnessconsulting.ca/book_bonuses.html** to receive your FREE Eating for Energy empowering affirmations.

3 We're No Longer in Kansas

I simply cannot reiterate the value of proper nutrition enough. It is the essence of what gives us life. Take away our nutrients and you've taken away life. Having the proper information for healthy eating nowadays is essential considering the levels to which we are being bombarded with so many conflicting messages as to how to eat for optimal health, weight loss, disease prevention, and so much else.

For instance, if you're looking to lose weight, advertisers get you all hyped up to pick up the newest "fad" diet book or instruct you to severely restrict your intake of carbohydrates. Proteins are good – carbs are bad. That's what they tell you! This is a message that has plagued our society over the last two decades thanks to the widespread acceptance of Atkins and other high protein diets. As you can probably tell, I'm not a fan of these approaches to eating at all. They are an abomination and frankly make me sick to my stomach! In fact, the healthiest and longest living cultures in the world follow a diet that is high in quality carbohydrates!

What I will be presenting to you in this book is a new way of eating that is really an old way of eating. It is truly the way nature intended for you to eat. I will get into much greater detail later on, but to wet your appetite, let it be known that you will be introduced to a nutritional philosophy that is little, if ever, talked about, which is a shame because it is so absolutely critical in order to maximize your health, performance, lifespan, energy, and so much more.

No matter if you're a couch potato, a high performance athlete, a type II diabetic, a cancer patient, or simply looking for better health, this approach to nutrition will dramatically improve your current situation. This is so because these eating principles are based on millions of years of proven success. This natural approach to food has been in existence since the beginning of time but unfortunately within the last two centuries it has been sadly overshadowed by the industrialization and commercialization of our food supply.

In science there is a principle called **Occam's razor**. This principle tells us that, amongst competing theories, the simplest is most likely to be true. Eating foods that are whole, natural, and living is simplicity. It is the way nature was designed.

If we were put on this planet with gas barbecues and microwaves right from the start, then I would probably not be writing this book. However, the simplicity and beauty of the earth's natural "fruits" cannot be overlooked. All the nutrition we will ever need can be found in the original state in which nature has provided it.

One of the major issues facing Western society is the almighty dollar, the quest for which is the reason our food supply has been absolutely ravaged. Food companies spend millions upon millions of dollars "creating" foods that save you time while promising ultimate nutrition. They like to trick you into thinking that because they're accommodating the latest trends (ie. eliminating trans-fats) that their foods are tremendously beneficial to your body.

I cannot help but laugh at a recent television commercial from a well-known American fast food restaurant that proudly boasts they no longer use trans-fats in their "deep frying" process. Who cares? It doesn't mean that all of a sudden their deep fried food is any healthier. You need to wake up and smell the roses my friend! You must avoid being fooled into believing what large food and drug corporations tell you. I may sound a little extreme, but if you knew what I do, I am sure you would agree.

In general, **my rule of thumb is to avoid any food or brand that is advertised – period!**

Stay true to yourself. Stay true to what nature intended.
To make matters even worse is that commercial farmers have been overtaxing our once "mineral rich" soils in order to achieve greater crop yields. It's not so much the farmers, but the large conglomerates that control every part of the food cycle and therefore

dictate farmer actions. The end result – even the healthiest of organic foods are dramatically depleted in mineral content compared with what those same foods would have contained 50 years ago. As an example, it has been estimated that broccoli, a vegetable which everyone knows to be healthy, has on average 50% less calcium and other important minerals compared to just 50 years ago. The pivotal **Earth Summit at Rio de Janeiro** in 1992 revealed some scary statistics pertaining to the declining mineralization of the earth's soils over the last 100 years. The scientists at this summit showed that the soils around the world have been dramatically stripped of the majority of their minerals. Here are some of their findings:

Soil Mineral Depletion Over 100 Years

(Earth Summit at Rio de Janeiro, 1992)

Continent	% Depleted Minerals Over Last 100 Years
North America	85%
South America	76%
Asia	76%
Africa	74%
Europe	72%
Australia	55%

This table shows that our soils have nowhere near the nutrient quality that they possessed just 100 years ago! And since our foods derive their nutrients from the soil, they are obviously compromised as well.

Look at the following chart to see how our foods have changed:

Changes in Mineral Content of Vegetables, Fruits, and Meat (1940 – 1991)

Year of Analysis	Mineral	Vegetables (27 varieties)	Fruits (17 varieties)	Meat (10 cuts)
1940	Sodium			
1991	Sodium	Less 49%	Less 29%	Less 30%
1940	Potassium			
1991	Potassium	Less 16%	Less 19%	Less 16%
1940	Phosphorus			
1991	Phosphorus	Plus 9%	Plus 2%	Less 28%
1940	Magnesium			
1991	Magnesium	Less 24%	Less 16%	Less 10%
1940	Calcium			
1991	Calcium	Less 46%	Less 16%	Less 41%
1940	Iron			
1991	Iron	Less 27%	Less 24%	Less 54%
1940	Copper			
1991	Copper	Less 76%	Less 20%	Less 24%

It is evident that our soils and food supply have been ravaged. However, by choosing organic foods you can help ensure that you get more minerals than from conventionally farmed foods. Organic farming practices promote greater soil quality and greater mineralization of grown foods.

I know that the above information paints a rather gloomy picture but it just goes to show that there has never been a greater time in history to ensure that quality living foods enter your body. You need to nourish your body with the healthiest possible foods to look and feel your absolute best and ensure you live a long and vital life! Being lazy is not an excuse. Choosing foods that have been boxed, bottled, or packaged is not an option. Yes, they are convenient, but the problem is straightforward - our body simply cannot handle and process the present-day "pseudo" foods we are currently feeding it.

Unfortunately, or perhaps fortunately, evolution takes a long time; hundreds of thousands or even millions of years. In your body's mind, you are still a caveman (or cavewoman) who is supposed to be feeding on natural whole foods. How is your body, which is an absolutely amazing machine by the way, supposed to know what to do with foods that have been processed, microwaved, chemically altered, fabricated, refined, pasteurized, homogenized, and cooked?

Your body is perfect. It was designed to be able to meet the needs and demands of nature. If you feed your body a wonderful apple, it says *"Thank you very much, I'll take these nutrients and put them here, I'll use these enzymes for this, I'll put these sugar molecules over here"*, and so forth. However, let's say you decide to eat some type of altered variation of this apple, for instance, apple chips that have been heated and injected with chemical preservatives. Now, your body is saying *"I'm not to sure what this is"* or *"I might recognize this particular molecule but it seems different, why won't it fit?"* The point is this - your body doesn't recognize foods that have been tampered with by human intervention.

It's like the Jurassic Park phenomenon where man decides to play God and things go horribly wrong. Well, things have gone horribly wrong. It is more important to your health than ever to eat according to what nature intended.

How a Stressful Lifestyle and Contaminated Environment has Made us Sick

Look around you. What do you see? Most likely you see people who are stressed out. They're running to catch the subway before the doors close or they're cursing as they sit in endless traffic. They're overworked and underpaid. In fact, they're not doing what they love to do, and they don't even know what that is! They don't sleep properly and require a liter of coffee to start their day. The list goes on and on...

It is evident that our lifestyle has become increasingly stressful. Stress is implicated in every single disease and illness known to human-kind. It is the common thread in cardiovascular disease, cancer, diabetes, auto-immune diseases, and on and on.

Stress can come in many different forms. There is the obvious emotional or mental stress described above. There are also physical and physiological stresses which arise from overexertion and undernourishment. For instance, if you've never exercised before and all of a sudden embark upon running a marathon, you'll put your body into complete shock! That is a stressor. You need to ease into it and allow your body to adapt.

How about if you eat poor quality foods? That too is a stressor on your body.

Our environment is also a stressor. Consider the polluted air we breathe, the contaminated water most of us drink, and the chemicals we use to clean both our clothes and our homes. I'm sure you can think of plenty of others.

My goal is not to scare you, but inform you as to what is happening to your body. Stress is all around you, so you need to do the best you can to minimize it and protect yourself.

So what exactly does stress do to your body? Stress has many negative effects, largely regulated by the action of the adrenal glands. The adrenal glands produce hormones such as cortisol, adrenaline, aldosterone, and the sex hormones.

In a state of acute stress, your body's first response is a quick signal to the adrenal glands to secrete cortisol and adrenaline. These hormones mobilize energy reserves (ie. glucose, fatty acids, etc...) and prepare you to deal with or run away from the situation at hand. This is known as the "fight or flight" response. You must realize that any stress encountered by the body will be perceived as if we were living hundreds of thousands of years ago – we have not evolved to deal with the situation differently.

In ancient times, when our Neanderthal ancestors encountered a dangerous animal, a shortage of food, or any other "survival" type of situation, this is how the body reacted so they could hunt, run, find food, and simply survive when times were hard. To this day the body responds the same way. Even though you will most likely never encounter a predatory lion in your lifetime, you still exhibit this "fight or flight" response to every single stressor in your life! The key is to learn how to manage and control your stress; otherwise, it will be your demise.

In the 1930s, the famous endocrinologist **Hans Selye** coined the term *GAS* or *General Adaptation Syndrome* to describe the process the body undergoes under chronic stress.

In a nutshell, this is how it works:

1. **Alarm Reaction** – In the first stage of GAS the body releases adrenaline, cortisol and a variety of other physiological mechanisms to combat any perceived stress and stay in control. This is called the *fight or flight response*. The muscles tense, the heart beats faster, the breathing and perspiration increases, the eyes dilate, and the stomach may clench. Believe it or not, this is done by nature to protect you in case something bad happens. Once the cause of the stress is removed, the body will go back to normal.

2. **Adaptation Phase** – If the cause for the stress is not removed, GAS goes to its second stage called **resistance** or **adaptation**. This is the body's response to long term protection. The adrenal glands secrete further hormones that increase blood

sugar levels to sustain energy and raise blood pressure. Overuse of this phase of the defense mechanism will eventually lead to disease. In this stage, an enlargement of the adrenal glands are noticeable as they try to keep up the on-going demands of stress.

If this adaptation phase continues for a prolonged period of time without periods of relaxation and rest to counterbalance the stress response, sufferers become prone to fatigue, concentration lapses, irritability and lethargy as the effort to sustain arousal slides into negative stress.

3. **Exhaustion** - In this final stage, the body has run out of its reserve of body energy and immunity. Mental, physical and emotional resources suffer heavily. The body experiences "adrenal exhaustion". The blood sugar levels decrease as the adrenals become depleted and shrink in size, leading to decreased stress tolerance, progressive mental and physical exhaustion, illness and collapse.

Research findings indicate that stress and depression have a negative effect on the immune system. Continually high levels of cortisol, the body's main stress hormone will lead to the suppression of the immune system through increased production of interleukin-6, an immune-system messenger. Reduced immunity makes the body more susceptible to everything from the common cold to cancer. For example, the incidence of serious illness, including cancer, is significantly higher among people who have suffered the death of a spouse in the previous year.

The far reaching effects of stress and high cortisol levels in the body are staggering. For the purposes of the book, we will focus on stress and how it alters your body's ph balance, opening the doors to disease.

In one word, stress creates ACID. Cortisol creates acid. Stress creates acid in your body and an overly acidic body can eventually lead to a plethora of conditions including sickness, low energy, weight gain, and disease, just to name a few.

To relate the effect of foods to stress, Maurer and his colleagues showed that the acid load inherent in the Western diet results in chronic high levels of acid in the body (acidosis) associated with a state of cortisol (stress hormone) excess. A diet more alkaline in nature helps to moderate the stress response and help the body return to homeostasis (balance).[6] What we have learned here is that a healthy alkalizing diet can help your body to better deal with stress.

Now that you know how much stress can harm your body, it is your responsibility to take the empowering actions necessary to reduce and manage it. So how do you go about reducing the acid load in the body? As you'll see throughout this book, choosing foods that alkalize and energize your body will have profound preventive benefits and help your body better cope with stress. Activities like yoga and meditation will also help, and I encourage you to try them.

---

[6] Maurer, M.; Riesen, W.; Muser, J.; Hulter, H. and Krapf, R. Neutralization of Western diet inhibits bone resportion independently of K intake and reduces cortisol secretion in humans, American Journal of Physiology and Renal Physiology 284: F32-40, 2003.

3 Action Steps

We're No Longer in Kansas

1. Make the decision to support your local farmers. Attend a local farmer's market, preferably organic, and get hold of the great local produce they provide. By supporting big business and their "criminal" farming techniques we only further the trouble in which we currently find ourselves.

2. Commit to spending at least 10-15 minutes with yourself each day in quiet meditation. Focus on what you want to create and visualize your life as you wish it to be. Stress only exists if you allow it to.

3. Take up an activity that brings you tremendous joy, be it walking, yoga, gardening, biking, or playing sports – whatever it is just do it. Having several physical outlets is a great way to lessen the stress in your life. Do your best to enjoy your activities at least every other day!

4. Don't worry about things that are out of your control. If you're stuck in traffic, don't fret. If you can't do anything to change the situation, then change how you perceive it. Stress is self-induced. Choose your battles. Worry and stress over things you cannot control will poison your body's energy. List 5 areas or situations in which you will commit to no longer waste your energy.

4 The Germ is Nothing, the Environment is Everything

To understand why the nutritional approach described in the book is so powerful, it is important to learn the basics of how your body works at the cellular level. We live and die at the cellular level!

To best explain how you operate let's go on a little journey inside your body. To begin with, I would like you to consider all of the arteries (blood vessels) in your body. The arteries are your body's highways for transporting blood, or your "river of life". Blood is what transports oxygen and nutrients to all of your body's cells while helping remove waste products produced in the cells. The blood is probably the most important tissue in your entire body – without it functioning properly, you die!

Within this "river of life" reside your red blood cells (RBC) which carry oxygen to the cells. Each RBC holds 4 molecules of oxygen; each one bound to hemoglobin (an iron-based protein carrier). These oxygen molecules eventually go to the cells of the body to provide the necessary input for metabolism.

From an electromagnetic perspective, (which I will discuss in greater detail later) each RBC has a negative charge on its outer surface and a positive charge on the inside. This ensures that no two (or more) RBC stick together – since two negative charges repel each other. This is absolutely critical to understand. Think about it for a moment - what would happen if all of the RBC started to clump together? Your blood would become viscous and sluggish, like thick sewage! Oxygen transport would be impaired and your energy would be reduced dramatically.

Well, what if I tell you that that exact scenario is taking place inside of you at this very moment, without your awareness!? That's exactly what's happening inside more than 80% of the population! Pretty crazy, I know!

Next, let us discuss the issue of pH balance and its role in the blood. First, a definition of pH and the pH scale is needed. The pH (potential of hydrogen) is a measure of acid and alkalinity and is measured on a scale of 0 – 14, 7 being neutral. A pH of 0 is very acidic while a pH of 14 is most alkaline. Your blood **needs** to be at a pH of between 7.35 – 7.45 for you to live. Right away you can see that your blood must be slightly alkaline. This is absolutely critical for normal enzyme function, oxygen transport, and pretty much every other process that involves the blood.

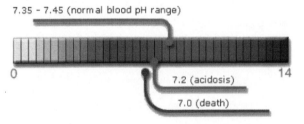

As I mentioned above, there are situations in which the negative charge around the RBC can be diminished or stripped. This can happen when your blood becomes too acidic. Too much acid in the blood strips away the negative charge around the RBC and as a result these oxygen carrying cells lose their ability to repel one another. So, they coagulate (or stick together) and your blood becomes thick, lethargic, and slow moving. Your body then becomes a reflection of this situation. You feel tired, lethargic, and sluggish. If oxygen and nutrients are not being properly delivered to your cells how can you be expected to operate at your best?

As these compromised RBC continue circulating in this acidic blood stream, they begin to lose their membrane integrity and leak their contents into the bloodstream – spilling toxins, bacteria, and debris. So, this "spillage" caused by the hemolysis (RBC destruction) further adds toxins and acidity to the blood; which in turn exacerbates the problem.

The Germ is Nothing, the Environment is Everything!

Each of us is at war and we don't even know it! The private war we each wage is a daily assault on our body by bacteria, virus, fungus, yeasts, and molds. Our immune systems become weakened and over-taxed in this war. Even the medical profession's first line of defense (the antibiotic) is becoming less and less effective against resistant new strains being created daily as the bacteria mutate. Since **Louis Pasteur** discovered the germ theory of disease stating that germs are the cause of disease, time has corrected him. Even Dr. Pasteur himself noted in his dying words: "The germ is nothing, the environment is everything."

The environment referred to in Dr. Pasteur's statement is now being called the *biological terrain* and comprises the body's digestive tract, lymphatic system, blood, urinary tract, and interstitial fluids. Our body is alkaline by design and acid by function – meaning that it produces acid as a function of metabolism. Maintaining proper alkalinity is essential for life, health, and vitality.

Under normal conditions, the millions (even billions) of microorganisms that reside within the body are generally not dangerous. However, an imbalance of alkalinity creates a condition whereby these pests can become pathogenic and promote the growth of bacteria, yeast and other unwanted organisms.

All leading biochemists and medical physiologists have recognized pH (or the acid-alkaline balance) as the most important aspect of a balanced and healthy body. They have long known that the maintenance of an alkaline pH in the tissues and cells is critical to cellular health. **Dr. Linus Pauling**, a 2-time Nobel Prize recipient, was the first to show that **cancer cells cannot grow in alkaline environments**! This is a very significant finding.

In contrast to the intended alkaline blood, the digestive tract (except for the alkaline mouth and small intestine) has varying degrees of acid by design, and the urinary tract should be slightly acidic for healthy function.

All of the cells (billions of them) that make up the human body are slightly alkaline, and must maintain this alkalinity in order to function and remain healthy and alive. However, their cellular activity creates acid and this acid is part of what gives the cell energy and helps it function. As each alkaline cell performs its task of respiration, it secretes metabolic wastes, and these end products of cellular metabolism are acidic in nature. Although these wastes can be used for energy and function, they must not be allowed to build up. One example is the often uncomfortable sensation of rising lactic acid levels created through intense exercise.

The body will go to great lengths to neutralize and detoxify these acids before they act as poisons in and around the cell, ultimately changing the environment of the cell. Most people and clinical practitioners believe the immune system is the body's first line of defense, but in actuality it is not. It is very important, but more like a very sophisticated clean-up service. The biological terrain (ph balance) is truly the first major line of defense against sickness and disease and for optimal health and vitality. Like stress, an acidic body depresses the immune system and reduces white blood cell activity.

If we were to ask "What is killing us?" the answer might be "ACIDOSIS"! It has been demonstrated that an acidic, anaerobic (lacking oxygen) body environment encourages the breeding of fungus, mold, bacteria, viruses, and disease.

Let's look at an example. If you were to seal the door to your freezer and then unplug it, come back and open the door in two weeks, what would you find? You will likely see mold, bacteria, and microscopic bugs. Things will be growing and multiplying. Where did they all come from? They did not sneak in - remember the door was sealed. The answer is . . . "they were always there". It is simply that the environment changed to a more inviting and "healthy" one for the critters to live in.

Another example is a garbage strike that occurred in New York City. With garbage bags piling up and a rotten smell mounting, a rat infestation came about. Now, would it be logical to say that the rats were the culprits in bringing the garbage? Of course not, the environment first became toxic and putrefied which then invited the rats.

This can be likened to a shift in your biological terrain from a healthy oxygenated alkaline environment to an unhealthy anaerobic acidic environment. **You see, what is healthy for you is unhealthy for the body's attackers and what is healthy for them is what is unhealthy for your body.**

A state of acidosis is simply an excessive build up of acid which causes a lack of oxygen. The blood is your body's first priority. If the blood becomes too acidic, your body will take the necessary measures to reduce its acidity immediately. Your body normally has alkaline reserves it can use to buffer excess acid in the blood. However, if you constantly pollute your body and create a chronic state of acidosis, these reserves will soon disappear.

How Acid Can Make and Keep You Fat

When your body notices that the blood has become too acidic and there are no longer any alkaline reserves, it quickly makes the decision to alleviate this dangerous situation. One of the first things your body does to alkalize the blood is remove the acid from the blood stream and send it to the fat cells.

This is critical to understand if you hope to lose weight. You can exercise all you like and will your way to a leaner body, but if you do nothing to alkalize your body, your attempts will be in vain. Think about it – the human body is very intelligent. As you become more and more acidic your body starts to set up defense mechanisms to keep the damaging acid from entering the vital organs. Acid gets stored in fat cells. After all, if the acid comes into contact with an organ, it has the chance to eat holes in the tissue. Fat cells and cellulite deposits begin to pack up the acid and keep it a safe distance from your organs. The fat may be saving your vital organs from damage.

If your body is acidic, it will require more fat to store the excess acid. Not until you start reducing the acidity in your blood will your body begin to realize that it no longer needs as much fat. So, less acid means less fat is needed to store it! Many people will testify that a return to a healthy inner biological terrain has helped them lose excess fat.

As mentioned earlier, stress is a big producer of acid. Consider the example of a woman who is obsessed with losing weight. It's all she thinks about. Do you think that might create some unneeded stress? Unfortunately, this scenario is far too common among women living in the Western world. An unattainable media and fashion portrayal of the "perfect" body has skewed the way many people see themselves. The result is that more and more people (not just women) are stressing about how their body should look. This type of worry or obsession creates greater amounts of acidity within the body and essentially works against their mission to lose weight. So, their weight goes nowhere and they don't know why!

Meat and Dairy = Acidity

Considering the acid-forming and disease-provoking nature of regular animal consumption, it is unfortunate that our society has placed so much importance on animal protein intake. Much of this "hype" has been a result of highly paid and very influential meat and dairy lobbyists (especially in North America). According to John Robbins, author of **Diet for a New America**[7], the National Dairy Council is the foremost provider of "nutritional education" in the United States! These councils and boards have tremendous influence as to what foods our governments endorse. They also have millions of dollars to spend on regularly running advertising campaigns. As a consumer culture we are easily influenced by what we see on TV and read in popular media print. This plays an important role in our decision making process. Just look back to the1980's when the entire low fat craze came to market. For some reason scientists and food manufactures believed that fat foods were making people fat. However, what we ended up seeing with the surge of low-fat and diet products was an all-time high in diabetes, obesity, and cardiovascular disease which stemmed from proportionately higher amounts of added refined sugars and other man-made chemicals needed to compensate for the lack of taste in fat-free foods. Unfortunately, we are still dealing with these issues.

---

[7] Robbins, J. (1987). Diet for a New America. H J Kramer Publishing; Tiburon, CA.

Recently Canada revamped its Canada Food Guide for the better. One of the greatest improvements is the recommendation that fruits and vegetables become the biggest and most important food group. However, foods from the meat and dairy categories still account for nearly 1/3 of an individual's daily caloric intake. You can see there is much room for improvement.

For many reasons, most being economical in nature, we have been brainwashed to believe that animal protein is a crucial part of our health. We've been told that if we don't eat red meat we're likely to develop iron deficiency anemia, B12 deficiency, and not get complete proteins from other sources. Most "fad" diets highlight the benefits of high protein consumption and recommend anywhere from 20-40% daily protein intake! That is preposterous!

Working in the field of fitness and performance conditioning I have been surrounded by many clients and trainers who firmly believe that they should be consuming their body weight (in pounds) in protein! Can you imagine that? I once worked with a trainer who consumed 300 g of protein per day! You'll soon learn why this can be crushing to your health.

According to the **World Health Organization,** only 4.5% of your daily calories need to come from protein.[8] The **Food and Nutrition Board** suggests that a 6% daily intake would be suitable to meet the needs of 98% of the population.[9] The **National Research Council** even figures in a substantial "safety margin" and states that just over 8% of your calories need to come from protein.[10] Coming in even lower is a report published in the **American Journal of Clinical Nutrition** which suggests that human protein needs amount to only

---

[8] "Protein Requirements," Food and Agricultural Organization, World Health Organization Expert Group, United Nations Conference, Rome, 1965.

[9] Food and Nutrition Board, *Recommended Daily Allowances*, Washington, D.D., National Academy of Sciences.

[10] National Research Council, *Recommended Dietary Allowances*, 9th ed., Washington, DC, National Academy of Sciences, 1980, p.46.

2.5% of total caloric intake. Many populations have lived in excellent health on this amount![11]

If you're not already convinced that we're eating too much protein, consider this: human breast milk, nature's perfect food, is only 5% protein. Cow's milk is roughly 15% protein content because baby cows need more protein! It is imperative that babies get the proper proportion of nutrients as the early years of life are the most demanding in terms of growth. Since we get 5% of our calories from protein in breast milk, doesn't that tell us that nature did not intend for our bodies to consume 20, 30 or 40% protein on a daily basis?

In most developed countries, the consumption of animal products is almost equated with status. There is a noticeable difference in animal consumption between socioeconomic classes as well as between 1st and 3rd world countries simply because of the cost associated with eating meat, decadent cheeses, and milk.

Unfortunately, the over-consumption of animal products has a direct and causal effect on our mounting ill-health and the degradation of our environment.

Years of research have demonstrated the acid forming properties and negative long term effects associated with the frequent consumption of animal products such as meat and dairy. This is one of the reasons that the nutritional approach in *Eating for Energy* does not endorse consumption of animal products. I must, however, be honest. I would be lying if told you that I didn't have the occasional piece of lean meat, mainly fish or poultry, once or twice per month. You may always be in a state of transition, which is entirely o.k. I encourage you to experiment and do what is right for you.

As you allow yourself to recognize the amount of suffering animals go through in the slaughtering process, the way they are injected with hormones and antibiotics throughout their lives, the way they are force-fed contaminated feed, and contained in

---

[11] Hegsted, D. Minimum Protein Requirements of Adults. *American Journal of Clinical Nutrition*, 21 (1968), p. 3520.

concentration camp-like farms, I would be surprised if you weren't less inclined to eat them. Not only are there moral/ethical issues, but the health ramifications (especially if the meat is non-organic) can be staggering.

If you are truly hung up on eating meat, then be sure that the meat eat is organic. Remember, you are what you eat. So if cows, chickens, and other animals are not being raised naturally, their meat will reflect their feeding, living, and slaughtering conditions. The intense fear that animals feel during their slaughter may very well add to the acidity inherent in their flesh, and be subsequently incorporated into your own tissues.

In 1995, a study published in **Kidney International** concluded that excessive dietary intake of animal protein resulted in a consequent increase in metabolic acid production resulting in mechanisms that lead to progression of kidney stones, bone disease, renal disease and a catabolic state.[12]

In 1997, a study in the **American Journal of Kidney Disease** stated that excessive meat ingestion and aging are two clinical conditions often associated with chronic metabolic acidosis. The body's response to this pathology is very efficient, which means that blood pH is frequently maintained within the "normal" range. However, pathologic consequences such as bone demineralization, muscle protein breakdown and renal growth are caused even though the bigger picture may look "normal".[13]

The link between meat protein consumption and osteoporosis has not gone unnoticed. Over half a century of studies have conclusively shown the detrimental effects animal consumption has on our bone health.

In short, the more animal protein you consume in your diet, the more calcium you will lose, regardless of how much you take in. The net effect is an increased risk of developing osteoporosis.

---

[12] Alpern, R. Trade-offs in the adaptation to acidosis, Kidney International 47: 1205-1215, 1995.

[13] Alpern, R. and Sakhaee, K. The clinical spectrum of chronic metabolic acidosis: homeostatic mechanisms produce significant morbidity, American Journal of Kidney Disease 29: 291-302, 1997.

The Acid and Osteoporosis Link

One of the body's greatest alkaline buffers is calcium. As your body becomes more and more acidic, one of the mechanisms it uses to regain proper pH balance in the blood is by calling upon calcium to maintain its alkaline balance.

Calcium makes up 1.6% of your body weight. It is literally the glue that holds the human body together. Calcium is so biochemically active that it has been likened to an octopus. A calcium ion can hold onto seven other molecules while it grabs onto one molecule of water. No other ion can do this. In addition, it is the perfect size to easily get in and out of the human cell, able to take a chain of nutrients into the cell and then exit to get more nutrients. It is a vital mineral for both bone health and muscular contraction, with many other vital roles throughout the body.

Earlier we talked about the importance of maintaining a proper blood pH. A compound called mono-ortho-calcium phosphate is the chemical buffer that maintains the alkaline level of the blood. Without it you would die. If the acidity level of your blood changes even slightly, you will die immediately. This is why I cannot stress the importance of alkaline foods enough!

In order to supply enough calcium to buffer the blood, you must have enough calcium being absorbed from your diet or your body will simply rob the needed calcium from your bones and teeth. Thus, when your body becomes excessively acidic it begins to leach calcium from your bones, which will predispose you to the development of osteoporosis. Not good! Many studies have substantiated these claims. Scientists have discovered that over time (and especially under acidic conditions) the human body becomes depleted of calcium. In 2001, research in the **European Journal of Nutrition** concluded that metabolic acidosis leads to greater loss of bone mineral and increases the potential for bone fractures.[14]

---

[14] Buschinsky, D. (2001). Acid-Base Balance and the Skeleton. European Journal of Nutrition, Vol 40 (5): 238-244.

Animal protein greatly increases the acidity of your blood. This not only includes meat, but dairy as well. Regular consumption of dairy for the purposes of calcium is absolutely detrimental to your health. Why? Let me explain.

First it is important to understand that the relationship *between* minerals is more important than the actual minerals themselves. For instance, the optimal calcium to phosphorus ratio is 2:1, a ratio commonly found in plant-based calcium sources such as sesame seeds and green leafy vegetables. Cow's milk, on the other hand, has a very high protein content which shifts the calcium to phosphorus balance to a 1:1 ratio. Upon ingestion, your body is then required to tap into its own calcium reserves to compensate for this mineral imbalance!

John Robbins, in his epic book **Diet for a New America**, highlights a particular study where young women maintained a positive calcium balance when their diets provided 1500 mg of calcium and 800 mg of phosphorus, per day. But when phosphorus intake was increased to 1400 mg, the women went into a negative calcium balance even though their calcium intake had not been reduced.[15] The lower the calcium/phosphorus ratio, the more bone density you will lose.

A landmark 12- year study conducted at **Harvard University** on 78,000 milk-drinking women found that those who had 3 servings of milk per day broke more bones than women who rarely drank milk.[16] A comprehensive meta-analysis of milk intake and fracture risk published in **Osteoporosis International** concluded (across 6 studies and 39, 563 men and women) that a low intake of dairy calcium (less than 1 glass of milk daily) was not associated with a significant increased risk of any fractures.[17]

---

[15] Hur, R. *Food Reform: Our Urgent Need*, Heidelberg Press, 1975, pp: 98-107.

[16] Feskanich D, Willett WC, Stampfer MJ, Colditz GA. Milk, dietary calcium, and bone fractures in women: a 12-year prospective study. Am J Public Health 1997; 87:992-7.

[17] Kanis et al. (2005). A meta-analysis of milk intake and fracture risk: low utility for case finding. Osteoporosis International, 16(7): 799-804.

If I've even got you thinking about why you may drink milk, I am happy. Remember, milk is highly acid-forming in the body. Here's another study showing the effects of an acid physiology on bone health.

A recent seven-year study published in the **American Journal of Clinical Nutrition** conducted at the University of California, San Francisco, on 9,000 women showed that those who have chronic acidosis (high acidity) are at greater risk for bone loss than those who have normal pH levels. The scientists who carried out this experiment believe that many of the hip fractures prevalent among middle-aged women are connected to high acidity caused by a diet rich in animal foods and low in vegetables.[18] This is because the body borrows calcium from the bones in order to balance pH.

Osteoporosis is very confusing for many people. Most people think they can avoid it by increasing their consumption of milk and dairy products. But in countries where the consumption of dairy products is very low, the instances of osteoporosis are rare. Conversely, world health statistics show that osteoporosis is most common in exactly those countries where dairy products are consumed in the largest quantities – the United States, Finland, Sweden, and the United Kingdom.[19] Osteoporosis is an acidosis problem. As the body becomes more acidic, to protect against the event of heart attack, stroke, illness, or even cancer, the body attempts to remain healthy. So, it steals calcium from the bones, teeth, and tissue. As bone mass becomes depleted, this is what we call osteoporosis.

As you saturate your body with calcium through healthy plant-based sources, you will raise your blood's pH (making it more alkaline) and reduce the acidity in your blood. This protects and preserves your bones, a giant reservoir for calcium since 97% of your body's calcium is stored in its bones.   If conditions such as acidosis are constantly present, those calcium reservoirs will be tapped into to bring the body back to homeostasis (balance).

[18] Sellmeyer, D. (2001). A high ratio of dietary animal to vegetable protein increases the rate of bone loss and the risk of fracture in postmenopausal women. American Journal of Clinical Nutrition, 73: 118-122.

[19] Jacobson, M. Preface to Hausman, P. in *Jack Sprat's Legacy – the Science and Politics of Fat and Cholesterol*, Richard Mauk Publishers, NY, 1981.

One of the first warning signs of an acidic biological terrain is calcium deposits. Calcium deposits come not from dietary calcium, but from the structural calcium of our bones and teeth! There has never been a scientifically proven association between calcium deposits in the body and nutritional calcium. Calcium buildup is also strongly linked to deficiency of magnesium, another important mineral that balances calcium.

If calcium deposits *are* forming, you will have an inner environment that is too acidic. Either your dietary intake of alkaline food is not keeping up with the buffering needed, or you are simply ingesting too many acidic foods. Either way, the result is the same: calcium will be pulled from your bones and teeth to make up the difference!

Meat and Cardiovascular Disease

This one is fairly evident. If you are or have been at risk for cardiovascular problems including high blood pressure, stroke, atherosclerosis, heart attacks, etc… , then I'm sure you've heard from your doctor to stop eating meat, especially red meat. Red meat is particularly high in saturated fat, cholesterol, and arachidonic acid – all of which wear down the integrity of the heart and blood vessels. Furthermore, if meat is from non-organic sources, then it has most likely been subjected to the injection of hormones and antibiotics. This is done to prevent disease in cattle and to optimize their growth. However, I'm sure you can appreciate that these "additives" are not healthy for your body. Remember you are not just what you eat. You are also what your dinner has previously eaten! As far back as 1961, The Journal of the American Medical Association estimated that 97% of heart disease could be prevented by a vegetarian diet!

Meat, Acidity and the Athlete's Performance

I've worked with so many athletes, both recreational and professional, that hold the belief that meat consumption is absolutely critical to their ability to perform, build muscle, and recover from training. Well, guess what? That's complete and utter nonsense. Since adopting a practically vegan diet, my performance, strength, endurance, energy, and ability to recover have never been better. Nowadays, I can easily get two workouts per day into my schedule without feeling the draining effects I once felt when I was a pro athlete eating high amounts of lean meat and refined carbohydrates. Although I no longer compete professionally, I still maintain a very demanding and competitive approach to my training.

If you are an athlete and are interested in performing your best ever, don't just take my advice, get inspired from some other real life athletic examples.

In a study published in the **Yale Medical Journal**, Professor Irving Fisher conducted a study in which he compared the strength and stamina of meat-eating athletes versus that of vegetarian (both athletic and sedentary) individuals. What the study concluded was that of the 3 groups tested (meat-eating athletes, vegetarian athletes, and vegetarian sedentary subjects) the vegetarians' (including the sedentary group) average stamina was double that of the athletic meat-eaters. There is strong evidence that a meat-less diet is conducive to greater endurance.[20]

Similar results have been demonstrated by several studies including that of Dr. Ioteyko from the **Academie de Medicine de Paris**, in which vegetarian athletes averaged 2 to 3 times more stamina and required one-fifth the time to recover from exhaustion compared to their meat eating rivals![21]

Can you begin to see what's happening here? As meat consumption adds to an athlete's already acidic body (from lactic acid production and physical and emotional stress of the given activity), the body is not able to spend its energy on replenishing and rejuvenating the body. The body must first alkalize the blood and then get the rest of the body back to homeostasis. This is all a big waste of time! If you can give your body a helping hand by alkalizing and energizing it through proper foods, why not give it a little help!? Remember, your body's first order of business is keeping the blood pH in that 7.35-7.45 range. If it deviates above or below that, extra energy and time will be needed to

---

[20] Fisher, I. (1907). The influence of flesh eating on endurance. Yale Medical Journal, 13(5): 205-221.

[21] Ioteyko, J et al. Enquete scientifique sur les vegetarians de Bruxelles, Henri Lamertin, Brussels, p. 50.

bring it back into balance. This means that your body will be able to spend less of its energy on the task at hand (ie. performance and regeneration).

More and more, athletes in every sport are realizing that a plant-based diet is the best way to fuel their bodies and help them excel. To name just a few:

World Champion gymnast **Dan Milman**
"Mr. International" bodybuilding winner **Andreas Cahling**
Tennis great **Martina Navratilova**
Olympian **Carl Lewis**
Football Hall-of-Famer **Art Still**
Four-time "Mr. Universe" title-holder **Bill Pearl** (described in more detail later)
Swimming World Record Holder **Bill Pickering**
World Class marathoner **Gail Olinekova**
Canadian champion tri-athlete **Brendan Brazier**

What are you feeding your body?

Is Cholesterol Really the Culprit in Atherosclerosis?

Just imagine for a second what would happen if you took an acidic solution and ran it through your blood vessels. Can you appreciate that there might be some damage that would occur? Well, this is one of the mechanisms that may lead to the development of atherosclerosis (hardening of the arteries), a precursor to many other serious cardiovascular problems.

We've established that acid in the blood can damage the blood vessels. Imagine the inside of your blood vessels being cut – almost like cutting your finger with a knife. Your body, being the amazing healer that it is, has built-in repair mechanisms for such occurrences. Usually, when you have a cut, a fibrin clot will lay down a meshwork of tissue to close the wound and new collagen will form over the cut so it can heal. This is how you develop a scab.

Interestingly enough, a very similar process occurs within your blood vessels. Your blood vessels like to have a constant, unimpeded, smooth blood flow. When damage occurs, the body sends its clotting factors, platelets, and fibrin to repair the damage. However, in most cases this repair process ends up leaving a scab in the interior (lumen) of the blood vessel. Because blood wants to flow in a smooth manner, the body searches within for a substance that will smooth over this newly formed scab in the vessel to allow for better blood flow.

Guess what it finds? Cholesterol! Yes, that's right. Cholesterol is brought into the troubled area to provide a smooth coating over the jagged scab. The trouble arises when this process repeats itself several times over resulting in a build up of cholesterol or plaque formation. This is the body's normal defense mechanism to heal a wound within the blood vessels. Thus, cholesterol is not really the culprit in the development of atherosclerosis. This wonderful molecule is incredibly important for your body's cell membranes, the production of sex hormones, and is an active component of bile (which emulsifies fat).

So really, the focus needs to be on preventing this cascade of events which causes vascular damage and cholesterol build-up in the arteries. You see, if you improve your body's alkalinity, you can provide a healthier cardiovascular platform for normal function and disease prevention. When it comes to heart disease, usually the first symptom is a heart attack! Cardiovascular disease is like a sleeping giant because there are no symptoms until it's too late. Your arteries need an 80% blockage for any symptoms to be detected! In most cases, by the time the blockage has been identified, major damage has already taken place as a result of hypoxia (lack of oxygen) to vital heart tissue.

"There are no specific diseases, only specific disease conditions, and there is only one disease. And that one disease is acidosis."

- unknown

As your biological terrain's oxygen level drops, you will begin to feel tired and fatigued, and fungus, mold, parasites, bad bacteria, and viral infections will flourish and gain a hold throughout the body. Often, you won't have just a few of these invaders. For example, if you have Candidiasis (overgrowth of *Candida Albicans*) you will likely have other bad bacteria, fungus, and parasites throughout your body because they all flourish in the same acidic environments.

The more acidic you become, the harder it is for oxygen to be present and your biological terrain will become more anaerobic. Without adequate oxygenation, your cells cannot carry on their life-giving functions in a very efficient manner because biological chemical reactions need oxygen.

Life and death occur in the biological terrain, so reclaim your terrain!

Are You Overly Acidic?

Here is a simple test you can take to subjectively assess whether you are too acidic. Answering YES to more than 5 of the following symptoms could indicate that your body may be too acidic and in need of alkalinity.

Lifestyle Markers

- I do not feel the best when I eat fast foods, fried foods, colas or desserts
- I do not feel my best when I eat red meat or red meat dishes
- I do not tolerate acidic condiments like vinegar or red meat dishes
- I regularly consume processed and refined foods that contain chemical additives.
- I regularly consume breads and baked goods made with white flour and sugar.
- I eat few fruits and vegetables.
- I drink more than one cup of coffee or tea a day
- I frequently take Vitamin C, aspirin or antibiotics.
- I do not tolerate alcohol

- I have a history of cigarette smoking

- I frequently travel by plane

Performance Markers

- I often feel exhausted after vigorous exercise or work

- I often experience low energy, fatigue or lack of stamina

- I run out of breath when running up stairs or walking briskly

- I am physically and mentally tired after an hour of desk work

- I am pessimistic, with little initiative

Physical Markers

- I have thin, porous bones

- I have poorly developed muscles

- I often experience muscle stiffness and soreness

- I am over fifty years old

Medical History Markers

- I catch colds and flu frequently

- I am susceptible to heartburn, canker cores, food and environmental allergies, and sore throats

4 Action Steps

The Germ is Nothing, the Environment is Everything

1. Go to your local drug store and buy a litmus paper kit (they only cost few dollars). Take a strip of litmus and place it on your tongue to test the pH of your saliva. The reading you're looking for is roughly 6.5-7.0. Even though this is slightly acidic don't worry as your saliva is naturally slightly acidic.

2. If you have the opportunity and resources I would highly recommend having your live blood looked at through a process called **Live Cell Microscopy**. You will actually look at your blood under a microscope in its living state. It is a very powerful eye opening experience.

5 Enzymes...
Your Life Depends on Them

What Are Enzymes?

Enzymes are proteins that accelerate metabolic reactions in the body. They are involved in every single bodily function from digestion and thinking to heart function. The 3 main categories of enzymes are *digestive enzymes* (ones that work on food digestion), *metabolic enzymes* (involved in every other bodily process), and *food enzymes* (enzymes inherent in living foods). Enzymes are the key to life. Without them, you die. And because they are used up in metabolic processes, you must replenish them if you wish to live a long and healthy life.

Over 60 years ago, the famous **Dr. Pearl**, of Johns Hopkins University stated:

"In general, duration of life varies inversely with the rate of energy expenditure during its continuance. In short, the length of life depends inversely on the rate of living."[22]

Because enzymes and energy expenditure go hand in hand, enzymes need to be constantly replenished. The more you use, the faster you age and decay. So, the more enzymes you have, the better off you're going to be.

It's important to remember that enzymes are very specific to which substrates they act on. For instance, the enzyme **amylase** works on digesting starch but not protein, while the

---

[22] Dr. Pearl (1946) of Johns Hopkins University in *Enzyme Nutrition* by Dr. Edward Howell. Avery Publishing (1985).

protease and **pepsin** enzymes work on protein and nothing else. So this element of specificity is important when discussing the role of enzymes.

Why Are Enzymes Important?

Many of the intractable diseases have two causes. The chief culprit is enzyme deficiency from undernourishment. Enzyme deficiency sets the stage and predisposes the body to ill health. A deficiency of enzymes speeds up the development of cancer, heart disease, arthritis, premature aging, as well as many other conditions.

The second more highly advertised "cause" of disease consists of environmental culprits including x-rays, bacteria, carcinogens, tobacco, and many others.

Let us look at the enzyme implication in disease. Unfortunately, as scientific literature has illustrated, each of us is born with a finite number of enzymes. Contrary to popular belief, enzymes are actually used up after completing their functions. This can be easily understood using a financial analogy. Consider for a moment that you have an **"enzyme bank account"** and that this bank account has an opening balance of 1 million enzymes (arbitrary number) at birth. Now, as with financial health, it's not necessarily how much money you make, but rather how much you keep and make work for you that is important. Therefore, the goal is to make more frequent and larger deposits than withdrawals.

In his classic book entitled **Enzyme Nutrition, Dr. Edward Howell** illustrates the "enzyme bank account" concept. The goal is to make as many deposits via food (ie. food enzymes) as possible to offset any withdrawals. As a result, your body (specifically your pancreas) will not be required to manufacture as many digestive enzymes to digest food. This is vitally important. When your food contains enzymes, the digestive enzymes that would have been used to digest the food are permitted to act as metabolic enzymes and circulate the body! These metabolic enzymes will break down any disease processes and foreign invaders rather than having to spend their energy digesting. This concept of lessening the strain on your digestive system is one of the most powerful benefits of eating an enzyme-rich diet. This is one of the key features of the *Eating for Energy* nutritional approach.

Making greater enzyme deposits is also highly correlated with longevity. The more enzymes you bring into your body through living foods, the longer it will take for your "bank account" to run dry. When the account runs dry, so do you! Several studies have demonstrated lower amounts of enzymes in the elderly. This supports the notion that enzymes are used up as you go through life.

Research has also shown that the people who live the longest (upwards of 110 years age) tend to have hypocaloric diets. This means that they consume fewer calories than conventional protocols advise. Lifespan can be increased by cutting down caloric intake. This occurs because of the reduced stress on the digestive system. Less food stress means that fewer digestive enzymes are required. Instead, more energy can be directed towards resolving problematic situations in the body. People are eating way too much food these days, and it will cost them a lot in the end. By choosing to eat a little less now, we can enjoy a lot more food later! This sounds like a good deal to me. Except, what if you eat a diet rich in living foods?! You'll soon see!

The effects of prolonged caloric restriction on health and longevity in the context of an equilibrated diet have been examined in Japan. A study compared data from Okinawa (where the number of centenarians is several-fold higher than in the rest of Japan) with the rest of the population. The researchers found that the total energy consumed by school children in Okinawa was only 62% of the "recommended intake" for Japan as a whole. In the adults, energy intake was 20% less than in the rest of Japan, although protein and lipid intake was about the same. The rates of death from vascular disease, malignancies, and heart disease were only 59%, 69%, and 59%, respectively, of those of the rest of Japan. The study, however, concluded that besides caloric restriction, other factors, such as genetic and environmental factors, were important in explaining these differences.[23]

One of the main theories put forward is that by reducing caloric intake, we minimize the amount of oxidative stress occurring within our body. And, as mentioned above, when we consume less food, our body is able to spend more time and energy breaking down possible disease and repairing and rebuilding our cells as required.

Having said that, let's turn our attention back to the "enzyme bank account". When we ingest foods that are void of enzymes, we are in essence making withdrawals from our bank account forcing our pancreas to produce and secrete larger amounts of digestive enzymes. The more often this takes place the more we set ourselves up for low energy, digestive strain, disease, and a shortened lifespan.

Have you ever eaten a heavy meal? I'm sure you have, and if you're like any other human on the planet you probably noticed a dramatic onset of fatigue within about 30 minutes of completing the meal, right? When the digestive system is strained with excessive food, the body is required to divert up to 80% of its total energy to the digestion of that food. This can be a very exhaustive experience. How many other activities can you name that drain the body of its energy like a heavy meal?

How We Drain Our "Enzyme Bank Account"

The consumption of foods that are void of enzymes such as cooked foods, refined foods, and non-foods (ie. coffee, refined sugars, processed and fabricated foods, etc...) all place high demands on our pancreas to secrete more digestive enzymes. According to the **Law of Adaptive Secretion of Digestive Enzymes** put forth by Dr. Howell, the pancreas will produce/secrete only the amount and type of enzymes required to digest a particular food. For instance, if you eat a meal that is solely meat-based, your pancreas will secrete

---

[23] Kagawa Y. Impact of westernization on the nutrition of Japanese: changes in physique, cancer, longevity and centenarians. Prev Med. 1978;7:205-217

an appropriate amount of protease to digest the protein and lipase to digest the fat in the meat. Because of the lack of carbohydrates in this meal, there will be little to no secretion of amylase (which helps with carbohydrate digestion).

Dr. Howell has demonstrated this law by showing that animals eating raw diets have no enzymes in their saliva, but will begin to produce salivary enzymes when fed a cooked diet.[24] Dogs taken away from their natural raw diet and put on a cooked-food diet had enzymes show up in their saliva in less than one week. The opposite is true as well. When they returned to their natural raw diet, the frenzied enzymatic activity in the saliva eventually disappeared.

If you consume high amounts of enzyme-void foods (ie. cooked foods) then you force your body to spend more energy on devoting its enzymes to digestion and less energy on producing metabolic enzymes for other bodily functions!

The incorporation of more fresh, living foods into your daily meals will help you make more deposits into your enzyme bank account. For instance, fresh fruits and vegetables and sprouted legumes are great sources of living, enzyme-rich foods. We'll get into specific foods a little later. Just remember that cooking kills enzymes and life. Cooked food is dead food!

How You Can Make Deposits into Your "Enzyme Bank Account" for Optimal Health

It's very simple. <u>Eat foods that are high in enzymes</u>! These are foods that have not been altered by the heating/cooking process. Enzymes are very fragile and are easily altered and destroyed. Enzyme activity increases as the temperature rises but only until about 118° F, above which enzymes become denatured and destroyed. To get the full potency that enzymes offer you must eat whole, fresh, living foods. As an example, raw celery has

---

24 Howell, E. Enzyme Nutrition. Avery (1898).

greater enzyme activity than does cooked, steamed, or boiled celery. You can apply this rule to every food on the planet, including meat (although I don't recommend eating raw meat).

In addition to losing inherent food enzymes when cooked, many of its vitamins, minerals, and important phytonutrients are also lost. A study in the February 2007 issue of **Food and Chemical Toxicology** revealed that boiling broccoli and other vegetables of the brassica family (ie. brussel sprouts, cauliflower, green cabbage) for as little as 5 minutes leads to losses of 20-30% of their glucosinolates, which are vital cancer preventing phytonutrients.[25]

Another important consideration when talking enzyme potential is that enzyme-rich foods have greater life energy. Life energy (or life force) simply refers to the energy (not calories) that these living foods provide. Traditionally, nutritional sciences have viewed foods from a caloric perspective when referring to their energy. However, I'd like you to reconsider this concept and challenge conventional thinking.

To view an example of the relationship between enzymes and the life force of food, visit our website at **www.totalwellnessconsulting.ca/food-energy.htm**. The images you will find demonstrate the life force emanating from various foods – an absolute must see!

Everything is Energy; Therefore, Energy is Everything!

In 1932, Dr. Harold Saxton Burr, professor of anatomy at Yale University School of Medicine, demonstrated that plants, animals, and humans possess electromagnetic fields, or energy fields. Using sophisticated equipment, these fields were shown to represent the vitality of the living organism. Health and vitality of organisms can be determined by the radiance of their constantly fluctuating energy fields.

---

[25] Song, L. & Thornalley, P. (2007). Effect of storage, processing, and cooking on glucosinolate Brassica vegetables. Food and Chemical Toxicology, 45 (2): 216-224.

You must first accept that organisms are more than their physical components, then you can begin to appreciate that non-visible elements or "non-empirical" elements can have a profound effect on how you feel. In fact, they are a representation of how you feel. In her book entitled **Food and Healing,** Annemarie Colbin states that a whole living organism, or system

"is an aggregate of physical elements and parts, plus an organizing energy field that makes the separate parts cohere and establishes them as a system."[26]

To understand the concept of life force, you must realize that everything is ultimately energy. Everything in this world and everything in this universe is connected through an amazing infinite energy. Trees, houses, cars, animals, foods, cement, and humans – we are all energy. The only difference is that your energy vibrates at different frequencies than that of other living organisms and objects. This is often discussed in the realm of **metaphysics**, the study of the nature of reality.

Before the development of modern science, scientific questions were addressed as a part of metaphysics known as "natural philosophy". The term "science" itself means "knowledge". The Scientific Revolution, however, made natural philosophy an empirical and experimental activity unlike the rest of philosophy. By the end of the eighteenth century it had begun to be called "science" in order to distinguish it from philosophy.

Metaphysics became the philosophical enquiry into subjects beyond the physical world, and to this day is not well accepted by the masses because it is not measurable. The saying *"I'll believe it when I see it"* is a common objection many people have to metaphysical ideas and the acceptance of universal energy.

For example, can you see electricity? Of course not, but you know it exists don't you? Otherwise many of the things you take for granted such as lighting, TV, radio, internet, etc.. would not be possible. But you can't touch, see, feel, or smell electricity.

I'll never forget what a mentor once told me. He said,

---

[26] Colbin, A. Food and Healing. Balantine Books, New York (1986).

"The only difference between science and magic is our understanding of how things work."

These words will remain as powerful as they were the first time I heard them. I truly believe that as we evolve as human beings and become more enlightened, we will start to look beyond the physical and begin to accept the idea that perhaps *"we might have to believe things before we can see them"* and not the other way around.

As we evolve into more enlightened and spiritual beings we begin to appreciate that there is more to life (and to this world) than our physical bodies. The practice of yoga and meditation are becoming much more popular nowadays not only because they are lower impact options for strengthening and stretching but also because they are great media for connecting us to something greater than ourselves – universal energy. A concept of economics states that whenever we are in a time of "high tech" there is an increased demand for more "high touch". Considering the fast pace of our technologically inundated world, more and more people are searching for answers. They search for their purpose on this planet and look for ways to feel more connected to something greater than them. It all comes back to the connectedness of infinite universal energy.

Every living organism on the planet is made of cells. If you investigate deeper past the cell you will find that there are molecules, composed of atoms. What happens when you investigate beyond the atom? What do you find? There must be something. Conventional science says that there is nothing to be found, but metaphysicists and mathematicians will tell you that atoms and every single thing in the universe are composed of "energy". Atoms are composed of protons, neutrons, and electrons which are held in place and/or repelled by energy. As you continue to investigate deeper beyond these elements you will encounter infinite space which is also energy. Energy is what holds everything together – even us.

If you have a tough time grasping this idea, I highly recommend that you watch **The Secret** and **What the Bleep Do We Know?** These movies will help you understand the connection between your thoughts and your ability to manifest anything you want in life, simply because you are inherently tapped into the infinite energy of the universe.

So, what does this have to do with food? We have established that you are made of physical elements which are held together by a fluctuating field of energy. Therefore, you are electromagnetic being. You know this is true because if you were to stick your finger in an electrical socket (which I don't advise) you would get shocked, right? This is evidence that our bodies are great conductors of energy. This concept has been well established and is accepted as common knowledge in the study of the body and its physiology. For instance, the eastern science of acupuncture is based on energy meridians within the body. So if you can conduct energy from a wall socket, is it possible that you can conduct energy from food?

YES!

It is important to realize that everything going on around you can influence your energy field. Food, stress, someone else's perception of you, atmospheric pressure, and cooking and food preparation methods will influence you – and the list goes on. You are affected by everything that surrounds you and you shape and affect the world around you as well.

Energize Through Food!

I'm not concerned with the details of how many calories are derived from various foods. I don't believe that is an effective approach when looking at what food can do for you. The philosophy of **Eating for Energy** revolves around consuming a living, plant-based, whole foods diet. This means that as much as possible you want to be eating foods in their whole state. For instance, if you need more vitamin C, it is much more beneficial to eat an orange or a piece of broccoli than to supplement with vitamin C. Our bodies were designed to recognize foods in their natural state, not their fragmented, synthetic components. Otherwise, we would have been put on this planet with supplements, microwaves, and barbecues right from day one. When you eat whole foods, you not

70

only get all of their macro and micronutrients, but you get these nutrients in their correct proportions. If you alter this perfect balance in any capacity you will alter the way your body processes the food (or supplement) for the worse. Simply put, fragmented foods cannot energize and nourish you as effectively as whole foods.

A great example is human breast milk which contains the perfect proportional nourishment for a young human. Per 100 grams, breast milk contains 1.1 g of protein, 4 g of fat, and 9 g of carbohydrate. This ratio is obviously what nature intended as the best formula for a human infant. Let's compare that to cow's milk. Per 100 g it contains 4 g of protein, 3.5 g of fat, and 4.9 g of carbohydrate. This too is a perfect formula but for a *calf – NOT* a human!

Many people swear by cow's milk for one reason or another, but when you consider that most cow's milk products have been fortified or enriched, further throwing nutrients proportions out of sync, it's no wonder we're dealing with so many health issues (i.e. osteoporosis, allergies, asthma, eczema) these days.

As human beings we are part of a global ecosystem. Each organism within this ecosystem subsists on what nature provides. Why should we be any different?

Fragmented foods are often referred to as "refined". An obvious example of this is white bread which has been fragmented by removing its germ and bran. But, since we are told that bran is important for our colon health, we then go out and buy a bran supplement to throw on top of our cereal. Why not just eat the whole grain in the first place?

So the message is this: keep it simple. The simpler you keep it, the healthier and more energetic you will become. Eat as nature intended and you will be better off than you currently are. Most people don't realize just how good they can feel. They tend to think "This is it! This is the epiphany of how good I can feel!" Well, I'm here to tell you that you have no idea of the type of health and energy you can experience. Just because you may never have felt the way I'm describing does not mean you cannot start. Start now.

You need to see food in a different light. You need to understand that everything you put into our body will either energize you or suck your energy.

Let's look at how this occurs.

Remember, every organ in your body works on micro-electricity, this electrical magnetic vibrational frequency made possible through your body's bio-chemistry. To "Energize" means to eat foods that are high in vibrational energy or that have great "life force". Foods only provide value when they can be converted into the elements necessary for this chemistry that allows electrical charges to continue.

Food actually gets to the organs through these little electrical charges. Are all foods equal in energy? For example, are all carbohydrates equal in the amount of electrical alive vibrational energy they possess? Yes or no? Your common sense knows the answer. No, absolutely not!

Again, visit **www.totalwellnessconsulting.ca/food-energy.htm** to see this magic in action!

Your goal is to minimize or avoid foods that take away more energy than they provide. Your body operates on a subtle electro-magnetic current. Nerve signals, the body's mode of communication, are electrical charges. Your brain, your heart, and all the organs in your body emit these fields of electrical vibrational current, and your cells communicate with each other through pulses of electricity.

As Anthony Robbins so eloquently describes in his **Get the Edge** program, once eaten, food is first broken down into food particles and then broken down further into colloidals. A colloidal is the smallest possible size of a nutrient particle. These nutrient particles are then carried to cells via electrical charges. If you eat something that is "lifeless" and void of electrical charges, then you're not going to get the energy that your body craves. The food itself will take more energy than it gives off. This occurs every time you eat foods that have been cooked, processed, fragmented, altered, etc...

Each of the organs in your body has a certain vibrational frequency of electrical energy (measured in megahertz) for it to function healthfully. The average of your core organs - your brain, your heart, your lungs – is 70 megahertz.

Food has the same measurable electrical energy. For example, chocolate cake has a vibrational energy of 1-3 MHz. A Big Mac has 5 megahertz of vibrational energy. So, if you need an average of 70 megahertz of energy, and your primary diet is made up of Big Macs and chocolate cake, you are going to be in an energy deficit. Your energy is going to be low. If your energy is low, will the organs of your body be working at their total functional peak efficiency? If they are not working efficiently, your organs will begin to shut down, and you will begin to build up more toxic waste. Your body would normally get rid of this waste, but your body no longer has the energy to function properly. This is the slow decline that most people would call "aging," and write it off as something out of their control. But as you now know, that does not have to be the case!

Let's take a look at some more vibrational measurements. Most vitamin and mineral supplements have energies of 10-30 megahertz – and that's if your body can absorb them. Raw almonds are 40-50 MHz. Your liver is 55-60 MHz; your colon, 58-63 MHz; your stomach, 58-65 MHz; the top of your head, 60-70 MHz; your brain emits 72-78 MHz. . Your body is basically in that 60-70 MHz range.

Green vegetables have the highest vibrational energy: 70-90 MHz. Live fresh wheat grass has 70-90 MHz. Plus, green vegetables are extremely alkaline! You want alkalinity, and green vegetables are some of the most alkaline foods you can feed your body![27]

[27] Robbins, A. (2000). Get the Edge – Pure Energy Live (CD). Guthy-Renker, Palm Desert, CA.

Feeding Your Brain

Dr. Howell also uncovered a very interesting connection between enzyme deficiencies (and thus energy deficiencies) in a cooked food diet and a decrease in brain size and weight.

In his work, he describes a study in which rats were fed a "factory" (cooked-food) diet. Their body weight went up and their brain weight went down. After reviewing the literature of over 50 similar reports, Dr. Howell demonstrated a significant relationship between a "dead" food diet and a decrease in brain weight.

It appears that food has a similar effect on your brain just like your environment and level of stimulation have an effect on the brain. It is well known that you are more likely to lose your mental capacity if you do not remain mentally stimulated, especially as you age.

This downward trend in brain weight may be due to the domestication of our brains. The brains of wild animals are almost always larger in size and heavier than those of their domesticated counterparts. The brains of wild meadow mice are twice as heavy as those of laboratory mice. Even **Charles Darwin** noted that the domesticated rabbit has a smaller brain than his wild cousin.

It is important that your brain remain stimulated. Wild animals are constantly stimulated in their environments. They must find food, shelter, and avoid predators. You too must stay stimulated through the performance of complex mental tasks and proper nourishment with foods that will improve its performance and prevent decay. It's a case of use it or lose it.

Proper nutrition is the basis of mental power. Negative thoughts of failure, pessimism, and despair are all associated with states of low energy and enzyme depletion in the body caused by eating the wrong food. It is amazing to experience the mental clarity, concentration, and creativity that emerge when energizing foods are consumed on a regular basis.

Brain cells derive nutrients from the foods we eat. Proper cell function requires basic building blocks such as essential fatty acids, amino acids, and vitamins such as choline. An enzyme rich diet is crucial in order to supply the enzymes needed for brain function, the building of neural networks, and the production of neurotransmitters. Just recently, the **Alzheimer's Association** predicted that the incidence of Alzheimer's will quadruple by 2050! Several theories have been put forth for the connection between food and Alzheimer's disease. For instance, there is increased risk for the disease in people who have elevated levels of mercury and/or aluminum, free radical damage, abnormal magnesium metabolism, and/or deficiencies of essential fatty acids and antioxidants.

We live by a sad but true irony. In today's world what we call "health" is really an incubation period for the development of disease! It's time to put an end to the madness. It's time to nourish and energize your body. The most critical element is that YOU HAVE TO START NOW! The best time to start was at conception. The second best time is now.

5 Action Steps

Enzymes...Your Life Depends on Them!

1. Challenge yourself to eat only raw fruits and vegetables for an entire day. Experience the difference enzymes make. Albeit this is only one day, you may set a long-term success path. Notice the difference in the way you feel. How is your energy? How do you feel emotionally? Do you have the same cravings?

2. Conversely, spend one day eating only cooked food (for experimental purposes only) and notice how you feel. Feel free to have whatever you like. You might notice that your body takes much longer to process these foods. Hmmm....it makes a difference when foods don't have any enzymes.

EATING FOR ENERGY

Living the Nutritional Lifestyle Success Guide

6 Creating an Alkaline Internal Environment

We've established with conviction that an overly acidic body is a risk factor for several disease processes, ill health, low energy, and compromised function across the board. Although this concept isn't readily discussed in most medical textbooks, it is an absolutely imperative reality to understand. Acknowledge that a healthy acid-alkaline balance is the key to optimal physical and mental performance and a healthy, long-lasting life. It is paramount if you are to move forward into making the commitment to greater health.

In order to get different results you must change your actions. If you keep eating what you've always been eating, you'll keep looking and feeling the way you currently look and feel. Do you want to feel better? I know you do! Who wouldn't?

In Western society, what we define as "health" is actually just an incubation period for disease. It's really only a matter of time before the majority or people succumb to diabetes, cardiovascular disease, or cancer. But not you! You've begun to take the necessary steps to alkalize and energize your body!

Most people don't even listen to what their body tells them. Feeling tired or bloated after a meal is not a normal occurrence of human digestion. These symptoms indicate many possible digestive issues. However, most people don't know how to listen to their bodies. Most people cruise through life eating whatever they want. They smoke and they drink without understanding what they are doing to their body's internal environment. My first piece of advice is **LISTEN TO YOUR BODY**. Your body will tell you what it needs. JUST LISTEN.

Where to Start?

So how do you go about alkalizing and energizing your body? How do get to that state of optimal health?

Follow the *"Eating for Energy* Food Spectrum"

The *Eating for Energy* **Food Spectrum** is specifically designed to drive more alkalinity and energy into your body! It promotes larger quantities of fruits and vegetables and supports your body with healthy fats and high quality plant-based proteins - all in their whole living state (raw).

By eating whole foods (not fragmented or altered foods) you will provide your body with the essential elements inherent in each food that your body needs for optimal performance. As mentioned in Chapter 5 (enzymes), the food enzymes present in living foods are absolutely essential to achieving the goals you're striving toward.

So what's wrong with eating foods that are cooked? Well, it's not the end of the world if you cook your foods once in a while but remember that the enzymes and life force are destroyed, and that cooking further leaches vitamins, minerals, and phytonutrients from these foods that are already lower in these nutrients compared to just 50 years ago.

The recommendation for fruits and vegetables from many authorities is 5-10 servings per day, yet only a small portion of the population actually achieves these numbers. Considering that most people only consume roughly half of the recommended number of these vital fruits and vegetables and that of this number the majority are contaminated (unless organic) and lower in nutrient content than in the past, we're at best only getting ¼ of what we really need. In fact, Americans are estimated to only be consuming 1-2 fruit and vegetable servings per day!

Cooking has never added, and never will add, any benefit to the nutrient value of a food. It can only alter it and make it less than nature intended it to be. From my estimation cooking only adds heat, some level of comfort, and slight flavour to certain foods.

Isn't it interesting that of all the animal species on the planet, human beings are the only ones that <u>need</u> to cook their foods? – Food for thought.

The *Eating for Energy* Food Spectrum philosophy is founded on living plant-based whole foods. Not cooked, altered, fragmented, or processed foods. The diagram below gives a pictorial representation of the *Eating for Energy* Food Spectrum nutritional approach.

The *Eating for Energy* Food Spectrum

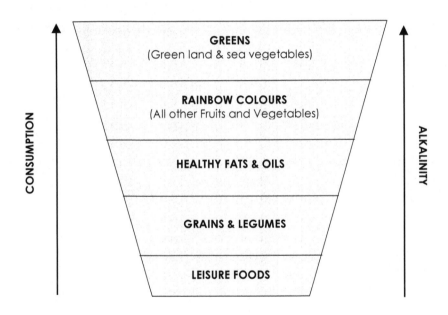

CONSUMPTION

ALKALINITY

GREENS
(Green land & sea vegetables)

RAINBOW COLOURS
(All other Fruits and Vegetables)

HEALTHY FATS & OILS

GRAINS & LEGUMES

LEISURE FOODS

Understanding the Food Spectrum

GREENS

This category comprises all plant-based foods that are green in colour (both land and sea-based). The GREEN group occupies the top part of the Food Spectrum because they are truly the most important group of foods available on our planet. Greens are the most alkaline of all foods and contain the highest nutrient density. They contain chlorophyll, the molecule that gives the plant its green pigment and which captures energy from the sun. Chlorophyll plays a pivotal role in the plant's production of energy (glucose and oxygen) through photosynthesis.

Chlorophyll is to plants what hemoglobin is to animals. Chlorophyll is the life blood of plants and only differs from hemoglobin in that it is bound to magnesium instead of iron. When you ingest chlorophyll-rich foods you directly take in the sun's energy and it radiates throughout your body. Green foods give you a direct transfusion of sun energy into blood energy.

Green leafy vegetables are the best source of highly alkalizing minerals: calcium, magnesium, iron, zinc, copper, sodium, and potassium. These alkalizing minerals neutralize the acid forming minerals (sulfur, chlorine, and phosphorus) found in nuts, seeds, onions, garlic, and animal products. Speaking of alkaline minerals like calcium, we are encouraged to drink milk because of its calcium, right? Well, where do cows get their food from? Grass! The grass is green and it contains huge amounts of calcium and all the other minerals just listed.

To further illustrate the point that we don't need dairy, here are some other sources of calcium from the green family. Keep in mind that cow's milk provides 118 mg of calcium/100 g and that the daily recommended intake (depending on the authority) is between 800 – 1200 mg of calcium/day. Therefore, to meet daily requirements and assuming that dairy is a balanced source of calcium (which it is not), you would need to consume at minimum 0.88 – 1.22 liters of 2% milk per day (considering 1 g of 2% milk = 1.1 ml)! That's four to five 250 ml cups of milk per day. That's insane!

Non-Dairy/Green Vegetable Sources of Calcium

Green vegetable	mg of Calcium/100 g
Kelp	1,093
Dulse	296
Parsley	203
Turnip Greens	184
Watercress	151
Broccoli	130

Source: Benjamin Barton. *Human Nutrition;* USDA Handbook No. 8; and Michio Kushi *The Book of Macrobiotics.*

Although green vegetables provide a great amount of calcium, sesame seeds are the #1 food source providing a whopping 1,160 mg of calcium/100 g. So if you're looking for a balanced source of calcium then look at having some more hummus (because of the sesame based tahini – see recipe section) and plenty of green vegetables.

The GREEN group includes (but is not limited to) the following green vegetables:

- **Leafy Greens**: kale, swiss chard, collard greens, beet greens, mustard greens, spinach, bok choy, watercress, mache, etc...
- **Herbs**: parsley, basil, coriander, etc...
- **Sea Vegetables**: dulse, nori, kelp, arame, irish moss, hijiki, kombu
- **Blue-Green Algae:** spirulina, chlorella

Greens also have the highest percentage of amino acids (protein) per ounce of any food. However, since greens do not weigh much, they need to be eaten daily to reap the full benefits that their amino acid profile offers. As you'll learn later, eating a large green salad and drinking green juice each day will help ensure that you get the amino acids your body needs to rebuild and strengthen.

Special Bonus: You can get an entire shopping list containing all the "energizing" foods in Eating for Energy when you visit **www.totalwellnessconsulting.ca/book_bonuses.html** to claim your FREE bonuses.

RAINBOW COLOURS – All other fruits and vegetables

Little explanation is needed to describe the plethora of health-promoting benefits that come from fruits and vegetables of varying colours. A good rule of thumb is to combine lots of different colours in your meals as this will ensure a wide variety of phytonutrients (i.e. antioxidants, carotenoids, flavonoids, etc.) that help to prevent and fight cancer and other disease (among other things). Furthermore, eating more fruits and vegetables will ensure that you meet your daily recommended intake of 35 grams of fiber. Fiber is so important for several reasons. It helps to improve cardiovascular health, improves intestinal motility and bowel function, helps you lose weight, stabilizes blood sugar, and gives you a sense of fullness. This is an abbreviated list, so just remember that fiber is critical to your health.

The RAINBOW COLOURS group includes (but is not limited to):

- **Fruits:** bananas, mangos, berries (all), dates, figs, papayas, pineapple, watermelon, mangosteen, persimmon, durian, apples, apricots, oranges, grapefruits, lemons, limes, kiwi, cantaloupe, honeydew melon, grapes, goji berries, avocados, olives.

- **Vegetables:** carrots, beets, sweet potatoes, broccoli, cauliflower, bell peppers, zucchini, cucumbers, lettuces (all), tomatoes, squash, mushrooms, onions, garlic

HEALTHY FATS & OILS

Many people fear fats. Why is this? I believe that most people don't understand fats. Most people think that if they eat fats, they will become fat. This is true to a certain extent, like when you consume high amounts of animal, rancid, or trans-fats. Without a doubt these fats will destroy your body and your health. As such, these processed fats have no place in your diet. They are not metabolically active and are easily stored as fat in the body.

Trans-fats are especially detrimental to your health. Trans-fats are fats that have been molecularly altered, usually by adding a hydrogen ion through hydrogenation. It is important to remember that these fats do not naturally occur in nature, so your body has no idea how to process them. Trans-fats increase blood cholesterol and LDL cholesterol (bad cholesterol). They have been linked to greater risk in the development of cardiovascular disease, cancer, and other degenerative diseases. Fats are needed to build cell membranes. When trans-fatty acids are assimilated into the cell membrane the cell begins to lose control over which substances enter the cell. Salt, carcinogens, damaging free radicals, and chemicals begin to accumulate inside the cell. The cell then becomes more susceptible to ultra-violet radiation, cancer, and other damaging forces. All research that shows the association between disease and fats has been conducted using cooked fats – not raw plant fats!

Healthy Fats are Raw Plant Fats

Conversely, healthy plant fats can have an absolutely amazing impact on your body and your health. Fats are required to transport fat-soluble vitamins, are a vital component to the cell membrane, and provide protection and insulation for your vital organs. Without fats we die! In fact, more than 60% of the human brain is made of fat. What makes raw plant fats so powerful is that they assist in their own digestion and breakdown! That's right! Because raw plant fats have not been processed or heated, they still contain their fat digesting enzyme **lipase** which helps digest these fats in the body. Therefore, even if your diet has a higher amount of raw plant fats, you are less likely to gain weight when compared to consuming the same amount, or less, of cooked animal fat. In fact, you will even lose body fat if you are following an adjunct exercise program. Furthermore, plant fats contain no cholesterol. Cholesterol is a compound found only in animals as it is produced in the liver.

Raw fats give you beauty! They make your skin, hair, and nails shine. Natural plant fats contain oils which lubricate the mucus linings and joints of the body. They are also beneficial in the alleviation of inflammatory conditions such as arthritis, colitis, asthma, bronchitis, and many others.

Some fats are called "essential" because the body cannot produce them. Linoleic and linolenic acids are essential fatty acids in which nearly all westerners are deficient. They are contained in the highly touted omega-3 and omega-6 fatty acids, which will be discussed in more detail below.

All fats and oils are composed of fat molecules called fatty acids. There are two methods of classifying fatty acids. The one you are most familiar with is based on saturation. There are saturated fatty acids, monounsaturated fatty acids, and polyunsaturated fatty acids. The second method of classification is based on molecular size or length of the carbon chain in the fatty acid. There are short-chain fatty acids (SCFA), medium-chain fatty acids (MCFA), and long-chain fatty acids (LCFA). All raw plant fats have LCFAs which help protect cell membranes from oxidation and free radical damage. Free radicals are defined as electron-deficient molecules. Raw plant fats (which have large amounts of spare electrons) help de-activate free radicals by giving them electrons! Essential fatty acids (omega-3 and 6) have a particular abundance of electrons and thus help in promoting optimal health and longevity.

Another term you will often see in reference to fatty acids is triglyceride. Three fatty acids join together with a glycerol backbone to make a triglyceride, so you may have short-chain triglycerides (SCT), medium-chain triglycerides (MCT), or long-chain triglycerides (LCT).

In a nutshell, (no pun intended) the HEALTHY FATS & OILS consist of fatty fruit, nuts and seeds, and plant-based oil. The healthy plant fats and oils that are recommended in *Eating for Energy* include the following:

- **Saturated fats**: coconut oil
- **Monounsaturated fats**: avocado, olives, olive oil
- **Polyunsaturated fats**:
  - **Omega-3s** - flaxseed (seed & oil), pumpkin (seeds & oil), hemp (seed & oil), walnut (nut & oil), fish oil
  - **Omega-6s** – sesame (seed & oil), grapeseed oil, safflower oil, sunflower (seed & oil).

Healthy fats & oils are crucial to your health, so I will spend some more time here to further explain the necessity and benefits of these fats in your diet.

Saturated Fats

These fats are solid at room temperature (except for coconut oil) and are very stable when heated which means that they don't become rancid (chemically altered). As such, they are safer to use if you cook occasionally. Because the philosophy of this book is based on living plant-based whole foods, no animal saturated fats enter the equation. The main source of saturated fat with our approach will come from the all mighty coconut.

Coconut Oil – the Undisputed Saturated Fat Champion of the World!

The vast majority of the fats and oils you eat, whether they are saturated or unsaturated or come from an animal or a plant, are composed of long-chain triglycerides. Probably 98 to 100% of all the fats we eat consist of LCT. Coconut oil on the other hand is unique because it is composed predominately of MCT (medium-chain triglycerides). The size of the fatty acid is extremely important because the physiological effects of medium-chain fatty acids in coconut oil are distinct from the long-chain fatty acids more commonly found in our diet. It is the MCT in coconut oil that makes it different from all other fats and for the most part gives it its unique character and healing properties.

MCT are easily digested, absorbed, and put to use nourishing the body. Unlike other fats, they put little strain on the digestive system and provide a quick source of energy necessary to promote healing. The digestive health advantages of MCT over LCT are due to the differences in the way the body metabolize these fats. Because the MCT molecules are smaller, they require less energy and fewer enzymes to break them down for digestion. They are digested and absorbed quickly and with minimal effort. MCT are broken down almost immediately by enzymes in the saliva and gastric juices so that pancreatic fat-digesting enzymes are not even essential. Therefore, there is less strain on the pancreas and digestive system. In the digestive system, MCT are broken down into individual medium-chain fatty acids (MCFA). Unlike other fatty acids, MCFA are absorbed directly from the intestines and sent straight to the liver where they are, for the most part, burned as fuel much like a carbohydrate. In this respect, they act more like carbohydrates than like fats and thus provide a great source of energy for physical endeavours.

Eating foods containing MCT (ie. coconut oil) is like putting high octane fuel into your car. The car runs smoother and gets better gas mileage. Likewise, with MCT, your body performs better because it has more energy and greater endurance. Because MCFA are funneled directly to the liver and converted into energy, your body gets a boost of energy. And because MCFA are easily absorbed by the energy-producing organelles of the cells, metabolism increases. This burst of energy has a stimulating effect on the entire body.

Several health problems such as obesity, heart disease, and osteoporosis are more prevalent in those people who have a slow metabolism. Any health condition is made worse if the metabolic rate is slower than normal, because cells cannot heal and repair themselves as quickly. Increasing metabolic rate, therefore, provides an increased degree of protection from both degenerative and infectious illnesses. The MCT in coconut oil are highly metabolic and thermogenic, meaning that they rev up your body's metabolism.

Furthermore, two of the main MCFAs found in coconut oil, lauric acid and capric acid, are highly health promoting. These two compounds are big time anti-microbial agents and are helpful in preventing infection and illness.

Next time you go to the store choose an extra virgin coconut oil instead of butter or margarine (more on this later)!

Monounsaturated Fats

Monounsaturated fats are found mostly in avocados, olives, olive oil, durians, cacao beans, almonds (and most nuts) and their oils. The slight electrical nature of these fats allows them to split and bind with some toxins. Monounsaturated fats are less stable than saturated fats yet more stable than polyunsaturated. However, as with the latter, these fats (especially in oil form) can go rancid with excess exposure to heat, light, plastic and air. Therefore, when choosing an **extra virgin olive oil,** be sure to get one that is cold pressed and comes in a dark glass bottle. Store it in a cool dark place such as a pantry.

Polyunsaturated Fats

Polyunsaturated fats are dominant in the substance and oil of walnuts, sunflower seeds, flax seeds, cold water fish, hemp seeds, and most other seeds. They have a strong electrical nature which allows them to easily split and bind to, and eliminate toxins. Because of this property, raw polyunsaturated fats are the most healing of all fats for the body.

The highly beneficial omega-3s are a subdivision of this fat grouping. They are present in many plant and seed sources (listed above). I recommend the use of **fish oil** for its high potency omega-3 fatty acid content. "But Yuri, fish oil isn't plant derived!" Yes, I know. Actually, it is in a sense because many fish feed off blue-green algae which are the ultimate source of omega-3 fatty acids. Along with whey protein powder, fish oil is the only animal-based supplement that I would recommend, and for good cause. The reason I suggest using a fish oil supplement (liquid form) is that all omega-3s are broken down into two compounds, EPA and DHA, before being ultimately converted into helpful anti-inflammatory hormone-like compounds called prostaglandins 1 and 3. A healthy liver is necessary to convert omega-3s into EPA and DHA; however, it has been shown that most peoples' livers cannot perform this conversion due to being in toxic, unhealthy, and malfunctioning. Fish oils, on the other hand, already come in the converted EPA and DHA form and thus are much more readily utilized by your body.

If you decide to choose a fish oil, ensure that it meets the following 2 criteria:

- Comes from **small fish** – sardines, krill, herring, etc…
- Has been **molecularly distilled** – ensures removal of all toxins.

Because polyunsaturated fats are the most fragile and sensitive of all fats, they need to be carefully stored to prevent rancidity. They should be stored in a cool dark environment such as a refrigerator for best keeping and should come in a dark glass bottle. To further avoid rancidity, they should be consumed within 30 days of opening.

Omega-6 polyunsaturated fatty acids, in addition to being converted to "good," anti-inflammatory prostaglandin 1, can be readily converted to pro-inflammatory prostaglandin 2. And since Omega-6 is easily attained in our diet, I recommend that you focus on consuming greater amounts of omega-3s to ensure a healthier internal environment. Inflammation is associated with all disease, so you want to ensure that your omega-3 to omega-6 ratio is in favor of the "anti-inflammatory" omega-3 fatty acids. Fish oil, flaxseed oil, hemp oil, blue-green algaes, and walnuts are all very good sources of omega-3s.

GRAINS AND LEGUMES

Grains and legumes are beneficial to your health. However, because they are slightly acid-forming in the body, they should be balanced by alkalizing green leafy vegetables from the GREENS group.

The GRAINS AND LEGUMES group consists of the following:

- **Non-Glutenous Grains**: quinoa, amaranth, millet, buckwheat, brown rice
- **Legumes**: lentils, chic peas, adzuki beans, mung beans, soybeans

I promote non-glutenous grains because they are less irritating to the digestive tract and contain a much higher nutrient profile than typical grains such as wheat or white rice. In essence, they are really pseudo-grains because they (except for brown rice) are actually more closely related to the green leafy vegetable family than other conventional grains. They are also substantial sources of protein with protein content up to 30%.

The consumption of whole grains, such as quinoa, has been linked to protection against atherosclerosis, ischemic stroke, diabetes, insulin resistance, obesity, and premature death. A new study and accompanying editorial published in the **American Journal of Clinical Nutrition** explains the likely reasons behind these findings and recommends that at least 3 servings of whole grains should be eaten daily. Whole grains are excellent sources of fiber. In a meta-analysis of 7 studies including more than 150,000 persons, those whose diets provided the highest dietary fiber intake had a 29% lower risk of cardiovascular disease compared to those with the lowest fiber intake.[28]

Legumes are also a great source of plant protein, fiber, and heart healthy carbohydrates. In combination with leafy green vegetables, legumes will furnish more than enough amino acids to build a strong and healthy body, build your immune system, and reduce the digestive burden on your stomach.

---

[28] Anderson JW. Whole grains and coronary heart disease: the whole kernel of truth. Am J Clin Nutr. 2004 Dec;80(6):1459-60. PMID:15585755

The following chart shows the protein content per 100 gram serving of various plant-based foods as well as several animal sources for comparison. Notice how none of the plant-based foods have any trace of cholesterol! To determine your "supposed" daily protein intake (in grams) simply **multiply your body weight (kg) x 1.0** (athletes may need a bit more).

Vegetarian Protein Sources

Food	Protein (g/100 g serving)	Cholesterol (mg/100 g serving)
Soybeans, raw	37	0
Lentils, raw	28	0
Mung beans, raw	25	0
Pumpkin seeds	25	0
Walnuts	24	0
Sunflower seeds	23	0
Spirulina	60	0
Spinach	5	0
Watercress	3	0
Ground beef	24	90
Chicken breast	29	84

Source: USDA Nutrient Database: http://www.nal.usda.gov/fnic/cgi-bin/nut_search.pl

As per the promotion of living foods, grains and legumes (nuts & seeds as well) should not be cooked. Rather they should be soaked and/or sprouted! Sprouting/soaking is a wonderfully simple method of awakening the dormant enzymes and the full nutrient spectrum inherent in these foods. By soaking/sprouting grains, legumes, and nuts & seeds you begin the germination process. This is really the halfway point between the seed and the development of a plant and is the point at which the food is most nutrient dense.

In the dormant stage, a seed has enzyme inhibitors to preserve and protect it. If you were to eat it at this stage, your body would need to expend huge amounts of energy to break it down. As you soak it, though, the enzyme inhibitors are released and the seed's enzymes are activated. The seed springs to life with an abundance of energy, life force, enzymes, and nutrients. Even squirrels use this technique to their full advantage. Upon collecting chestnuts, squirrels will bury them deep in the soil for several days so that they begin to germinate. Once this has happened, the squirrel returns to dig up the "activated" and "alive" chestnut for consumption. Isn't that absolutely amazing?

By soaking/sprouting, you can often double and even triple the nutrient content of the seed while reducing the seed's fat content and converting some of its denser vegetable protein into easier to process amino acids. This is invaluable because it means that you can eat less while getting more from your food and save money on unnecessary groceries.

Soaking 101

Soaking is as simple as its name implies. All that is required is some good quality filtered or spring water and the seed, nut, grain or legume you wish to soak. Remember that when you soak dried foods they will absorb water, swell and expand, so make sure there is plenty of water to cover them. It is best to soak them in a bowl or glass jar. For simplicity, **it is easiest to soak the seed, nut, grain, or legume overnight in water at room temperature.** After you have soaked your seeds, nuts, grains, or legumes they should be rinsed off before consuming or sprouting them. Soaked nuts (and sunflower seeds) don't necessarily need to be sprouted. They can be enjoyed in their living state after their overnight soaking period. If you have soaked a larger quantity of nuts (or sunflower seeds), then leftovers may be kept soaking in water in the fridge for up to 48 hours.

Sprouting 101

Now that you have your grains, legumes, and seeds soaked and ready to sprout here's what you need. First, ensure that you've thoroughly rinsed them after the soaking process. Next, using a sprouting jar, sprouting tray, or even a common strainer, place your soaked grain/legume/seed inside and make sure that there is enough ventilation and that the temperature is not above 80° F. You can easily make your own sprout jars by taking a wide-mouth glass jar and covering it with some cheesecloth (secured by an elastic band). Tilt the jar at a 45° angle and place it in your dish rack so that water from your seeds can drain properly and to ensure the jar has good ventilation. I personally just throw my soaked seeds into a strainer overhanging the sink and cover it with a kitchen towel or paper towel. As the seed goes through the sprouting process, you need to rinse it once or twice a day to maintain its moisture. Depending on the seed/grain/legume you are sprouting different harvesting times will apply. To test whether the sprouts are ready, chew one. It should be firm, yet soft and not too crunchy.

Refer to the following chart for some guidance.

Sprouting/Harvesting Time Chart

Nut, Seed, Legume, or Grain	Sprouting Time
Adzuki beans	3-5 days
Alfalfa	4-6 days
Buckwheat, hulled	1-3 days
Clover sprouts	4-6 days
Green lentils	1-3 days
Red lentils	1 day
Mung beans	1-3 days
Peas	2-4 days
Oat Groats	2-3 days
Quinoa	1-2 days
Chic Peas	3-4 days
Amaranth	1-2 days
Millet	1-2 days

Once the seed/grain/legume has finished sprouting you may store it in covered bowl or Tupperware container in the refrigerator. Most sprouts will keep for several days but it's best to quickly smell them before eating to ensure they haven't gone bad.

LEISURE FOODS

I am firm believer in moderation, balance, and sustainability. I understand first hand that maintaining a strict raw diet is just not practical for most people. Considering most peoples' habits, minimal availability of quick-to-go healthy foods, and lack of practice with raw foods, many people find it difficult to maintain a 100% raw food lifestyle. However, for the sake of your health you seriously need to make a concerted effort. At the same time, I can appreciate the occasional splurge or indulgence is to be expected and absolutely understandable. My personal vice is pizza...and sweets. So that's why I've left some "flex" in this living plant-based foods approach. However, don't abuse your privilege. If you're going to have leisure foods, enjoy them in moderation.

What you'll most likely find after following the principles and delicious recipes in *Eating for Energy* is that you'll no longer crave "traditional" foods and even if you consume them on occasion your body will immediately feel their effects. As you adopt this new food philosophy you will be cleansing your body of many of the toxins that have built up from years of cooked food intoxication. As your body becomes cleaner, you will notice marked differences in how you feel and react to foods that were common place in your diet.

In my case, I grew up eating tons of bread, cereals, dairy, and sweets. To this day it is still challenging to turn a blind eye to these foods because my body has been conditioned to enjoy them. However, as I my diet has evolved to consist of about 85% raw plant-based foods, the urge or craving for these foods has dissipated. However, on the occasion where I indulge in bread or other wheat-based products, my body feels it immediately. The bloating, gas, fatigue all present themselves within minutes to hours. Is it really worth it? I'll let you decide.

Most often, the foods we crave are the same very foods to which we are allergic or sensitive. As you move away from the foods that have handcuffed and debilitated you for so long, you will feel empowered, in control, and happier. No longer will food be the boss of you. You were destined to be free and to live the healthiest life ever.

As human beings we have the potential to live well beyond the age of 100. We are in complete control of our destiny through the foods we eat and the lifestyle we adopt. The choice is yours.

So the LEISURE FOODS group is really to give you the choice and flexibility to enjoy some of the foods that you've typically enjoyed while simultaneously offering you the possibility to completely eliminate them. Just remember, it will be difficult to move forward in your growth if you're still dependent on foods that hold you back.

The key is to make your 80% living foods become your leisure foods! But even if you can't or don't want to, that's fine as well. The health and energy benefits you will experience simply by consuming more whole living plant-based foods, even it's only a fraction more than what you're currently consuming, will be dramatic. Obviously, since the LEISURE FOODS group occupies the lowest position on the *Eating for Energy* Food Spectrum, these foods should be consumed the least. For maximum vitality, no more than 20% of your meals should come from LEISURE FOODS – the rest should be raw and plant-based.

7 12 *Eating for Energy* Super Foods

Avocados

The avocado is the new world olive. It is the fatty fruit that dominates the Americas as the olive dominates the Mediterranean world. The word "avocado" actually means "testicle tree" in the ancient Aztec dialect. Apparently, it not only resembles a testicle and grows in pairs but it also greatly enhances sexual passion!

As with most fatty fruits, avocados ripen on the ground (not on the tree), are susceptible to environmental conditions, and pick up superior taste when grown in mineral-rich soil. Over 500 different types of avocados have been identified. Because of their healthy fat content and grounding properties, avocados (and other fatty plant foods) are a great transition food from a cooked diet.

One avocado contains approximately 300 calories and is packed full of super nutrients. Roughly 90% fat, the avocado contains mostly omega-9 fatty acids and monounsaturated fats. Avocados are a great source of B vitamins (except B12), and antioxidant vitamins A, C, and E. They are also rich in potassium, magnesium, iron, and manganese.

For vegetarians who do not eat a lot of fatty foods, avocados are a terrific source of healthy fats and oils and provide a feeling of satiety when eaten. As you'll see later in the recipe section, avocados provide a beautiful creaminess that forms the base of many soups, dips, and sauces. Sometimes, I'll even just eat an avocado with a spoon by halving it, drizzling some lemon juice and apple cider vinegar, adding a dash of fresh ground pepper and sea salt, and voila! Absolutely delicious – and nutritious! If you're worried about the calories then obviously keep your avocado consumption in check – don't over do it. One a day is plenty.

In his book **The Sunfood Diet Success System**[29], raw food expert David Wolfe shows that the avocado has the propensity to save the planet and the human race. He claims that replacing meat and dairy fat (resource-depleting and health impairing products) with avocado fat would save millions of acres of land. At least 260 million acres of U.S. forests have been cleared for cropland to fuel the meat-centered diet and 85% of U.S. topsoil loss is directly attributable to the raising of livestock. He explains that more than 50% of the water used in the U.S. is used for livestock production. It takes 2,500 gallons of water to produce just one pound of meat! Avocado trees, conversely, provide health promoting food, create clean air, enhance topsoil, and provide homes for wildlife.

---

[29] Wolfe, D. The Sunfood Diet Success System. Maul Bros. Publishing, San Diego, CA (2006).

Olives (and olive oil)

Like its trans-Atlantic cousin the avocado, the olive is a wonderful fatty fruit also touted for its aphrodisiac effect. In fact, many raw foodists claim that olives may very well be the world's most perfect food! In ancient Greece, Solon, the great law-maker, enacted laws protecting all olive trees and made it a capital offense to kill a tree or cut one down.

Olives and their oil contain some of the most beneficial fats – monounsaturates. Olive oil has been shown to be cardioprotective by lowering LDL cholesterol (bad type).

Consider the power and benefits of the amazing raw olive:

- Fruit richest in minerals
- Fruit richest in calcium. Contains twice as much calcium as oranges by weight.
- High in magnesium
- High in amino acids, including leucine, aspartic acid, and glutaminic acid.
- An alkaline fatty fruit
- Amazing source of monounsaturated fats but also loaded with omega-3 and omega-6 fatty acids.
- Great source of vitamins A, E, and many of the B vitamins.
- High in anti-oxidants
- Able to soothe mucus membranes with its oil
- The highest mucus dissolver of any fruit (figs are second)

When choosing raw olives, select ones that have not been soaked in vinegar as they are more acid-forming. Canned or pre-bottled olives should not even be a consideration as they are loaded with excess sodium, have been pasteurized, and many will have been soaked in ferrous gluconate (an iron compound which darkens them). If you don't have an olive tree in your backyard (most of us don't) and you can't find raw organic sun-ripened olives (best option), then choose olives that have been "water-cured", "sea salt-cured" and/or "olive oil-cured".

I personally enjoy olives as an extra topping on many of the raw pastas and salads that I make. I find they add a wonderful flavour and provide a greater sense of satiety after eating my meal. They are also great to use when making tapenades and other great dips or sauces.

Coconuts (and their water and oil/butter)

The benefits of this wonderful saturated fat have been described earlier on. However, I'll give you some additional information to help you incorporate coconuts and their oil/butter into your diet.

First, if you can get your hands on young coconuts then you can enjoy the wonderful white fleshy meat they provide. Young coconuts are easier to open then typical mature coconuts. The difference between the two is that mature coconuts have the traditional brown "hair-like" hard shell that you often see in the tropics. Young coconuts on the other hand are white, softer, and come with the husks trimmed down. They sit flat with a pointed top. I find that most Asian markets carry young coconuts. To open these young coconuts, a cleaver is your best option.

Here are some step-by-step instructions to help you get into your young coconuts:

1. Lay the coconut on its side, securing it so it won't roll.
2. Holding the knife high, bring it down sharply near the top of the coconut (be sure to keep your other hand out of harms way). The knife should sink in about one-third of the way, breaking through the outer shell.
3. Quickly set the coconut upright so you don't lose the precious water inside.
4. Drain the coconut of its water, then use the cleaver to finish cutting off the top to get to the meat.
5. The best way to get the meat out is by using the back of a spoon to pry it from the sides of the coconut, and then trim away any shell residue with a knife.

The water found inside fresh young coconuts is a natural sport drink - high in vitamin C, B vitamins, proteins, and electrolytes! Fans of coconut water rave about the beautifying powers that range from restoring chapped lips to combating the appearance of freckles, sunspots, and skin cancers! Young coconut water has also been shown to assist the function of the gall bladder, kidney, liver, and thyroid. What you probably have already seen in stores is "coconut milk". This is the extract of the grated flesh of mature coconuts, which generally comes pasteurized in a can, and thus would not be an ingredient that I would recommend.

When selecting coconut oil or "butter" it's important to buy only **cold-pressed extra virgin oil**, which is mechanically extracted from the young coconut meat. Be sure to stay away from hydrogenated coconut oil. This has been chemically altered (ie. trans-fat production) and is not healthy for you. Coconut oil will become liquid when stored above 24°C and will turn hard when stored in the refrigerator. I would recommend keeping it in the refrigerator for long term storage and simply placing its container in warm water thereafter if you want it in liquid form before using.

Spirulina

This is a true powerhouse! Spirulina is a type of blue-green algae that has been commonly found, amongst other locations, in Oregon's Klamath Lake. It has a very rich nutrient profile and is commonly used as a high protein nutrient because it contains all of the 22 amino acids the body requires. Per 100 grams, it contains 60 grams of protein! Because it is dark green in colour, it is a very good source of chlorophyll, is considered a rejuvenator of the body, and helpful in building healthy alkaline blood.

Spirulina is also rich in gamma linoleic acid (GLA), the oil found in evening primrose oil. It is possible that the GLA found in spirulina accounts for some of the positive effects of that people experience when using it such as mental clarity, improved energy, and a decreased appetite (weight loss).

Algaes, like spirulina, are the original source of omega-3 fatty acids. Algaes are what small, bottom feeding fish consume. These fish are then eaten by larger ones, and then eventually by humans. Cold water fish, which are well-known for their omega-3 fatty acids, owe their "omega-3 fame" to the consumption of algaes, even if indirectly.

Spirulina comes in powdered form and should be stored in the refrigerator. Ensure that you choose 100% raw, organic spirulina. I find that spirulina goes best with fruit juices and fruit-based smoothies. If you're a true warrior you can also just mix it with water but watch out for its peculiar taste.

Parsley

Parsley is native to the Mediterranean. While it has been cultivated for more than 2,000 years, parsley was used medicinally prior to being consumed as food. The ancient Greeks held parsley to be sacred, using it to not only adorn victors of athletic contests, but also for decorating the tombs of the deceased.

Parsley contains two types of unusual components that provide unique health benefits. The first type is volatile oil components - including *myristicin*, *limonene*, *eugenol*, and *alpha-thujene*. Myristicin, specifically, has been shown to inhibit tumor growth and helps to activate the body's most powerful antioxidant, glutathione. The second type of heath promoting component in parsley is flavonoids - including *apiin*, *apigenin*, *crisoeriol*, and *luteolin*, all of which are powerful antioxidants.

Parsley is extremely high in vitamin C and vitamin A (beta-carotene). It is also the greatest source of iron of any green vegetable! Another great feature of parsley is that it's a good source of folic acid, a crucial B vitamin which helps prevent heart disease by converting the "heart-dangerous" homocysteine molecule into its benign state. Folic acid is essential for many mothers-to-be, preventing spinal column-related birth defects in their newborns.

Whenever possible, choose fresh parsley over the dried form since it is fresher and superior in flavor. Choose parsley that is deep green in color and looks fresh and crisp. Avoid bunches that have leaves that are wilted or yellow as this indicates that they are either over-mature or damaged. As with any other food, try to select organically grown parsley since this will give you more assurance that the herbs have not been irradiated. Irradiation has become common practice in the sterilization of food. It involves exposing food to radiation in order to kill bacteria and increase shelf life. This process also kills vital food enzymes.

Fresh parsley should be kept in the refrigerator in a plastic bag. If the parsley is slightly wilted, either sprinkle it lightly with some water or wash it without completely drying it before storing in the refrigerator.

Cacao

Cacao (aka. Raw chocolate) is the seed of an Amazonian fruit tree brought to Central America during or before the time of the Olmecs, an ancient Mexican tribe. It is the main ingredient in chocolate. Cacao beans were so revered by the Mayans and Aztecs that they used them as money! In 1753 Carl von Linnaeus, the 18th-century Swedish scientist, thought that cacao was so important that he named the genus and species of this tree himself. He named this tree: *Theobroma cacao*, which literally means "cacao, the food of the gods."

Cacao beans contain no sugar and between 12% and 50% fat depending on variety and growth conditions. But rest assured there is no evidence that implicates cacao bean consumption with obesity! Remember that fat in its raw state contains lipase, the enzyme that metabolizes fat.

One of cacao's greatest features is that it is remarkably rich in magnesium. Cacao seems to be the #1 source of magnesium of any food. Because magnesium is a natural relaxant it could explain why women crave chocolate during their menstrual periods. Magnesium balances brain chemistry, builds strong bones, and is associated with more happiness. Magnesium is the most deficient major mineral in the Standard American Diet (SAD); over 80% of Americans are chronically deficient in Magnesium!

Cacao does contain subtle amounts of caffeine and theobromine. However, experiments have shown that these stimulants are far different when consumed raw than cooked. Consider the results from an interesting experiment that led homeopaths to indicate cacao's stimulating effect to be significant when cooked, not raw. The experiment, conducted with a mixture of roasted ground cacao beans in boiling water, produced effects similar to those caused by black coffee: an excitement of the nervous system, an excited state of circulation, and an accelerated pulse. Interestingly, when the same decoction was made with raw, unroasted beans, neither effect was noticeable, leading the researchers to conclude that the physiological changes were caused by aromatic substances released during roasting. I can tell you from my own experience that the energy you feel after eating raw cacao is absolutely phenomenal. And it doesn't produce withdrawal symptoms as you'd experience with coffee.

Cacao also seems to diminish appetite, probably due to its monoamine oxidase enzyme inhibitors (MAO inhibitors) - these are different from digestive enzyme inhibitors found in most nuts and seeds. These rare MAO inhibitors actually produce favorable results when consumed by allowing more serotonin and other neurotransmitters to circulate in the brain. According to **Dr. Gabriel Cousens**, MAO inhibitors facilitate "youthening" and rejuvenation.

Cacao also contains Phenylethylamine (PEA). PEA is an adrenal-related chemical created within the brain and released when we are in love. This is one of the reasons why love and chocolate have a deep correlation. PEA also plays a role in increasing focus and alertness. Yet another neurotransmitter, anandamide, has been isolated in cacao. Anandamide is produced naturally in the brain and is known as "The Bliss Chemical" because it is released when we are feeling fantastic. Cacao contains enzyme inhibitors that decrease your body's ability to breakdown anandamide. This means that natural anandamide and/or cacao anandamide may stick around longer, making you feel extra blissful when you eat cacao.

Many people have reported allergies to chocolate. However, is it the cacao or the dairy in the chocolate that is causing the problem? Well, a recent study showed that only one out of 500 people who thought they were allergic to chocolate actually tested positive. Allergies to cacao are quite rare. It is typically the case that the person is in fact allergic to milk and dairy products or some other ingredient in commercial chocolate.

Cacao has been touted as the number one source of antioxidants of any food on the planet! It blows blueberries out of the water. Antioxidants are measured using the ORAC or the "oxidative reactive capacity" of a given food. Have a look at the following ORAC chart (from rawfood.com) and you'll see exactly where cacao scores.

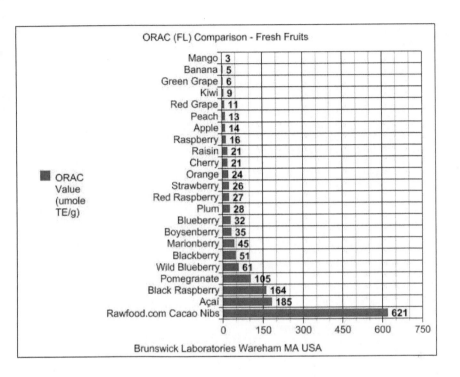

ORAC (FL) Comparison - Fresh Fruits

Fruit	ORAC Value
Mango	3
Banana	5
Green Grape	6
Kiwi	9
Red Grape	11
Peach	13
Apple	14
Raspberry	16
Raisin	21
Cherry	21
Orange	24
Strawberry	26
Red Raspberry	27
Plum	28
Blueberry	32
Boysenberry	35
Marionberry	45
Blackberry	51
Wild Blueberry	61
Pomegranate	105
Black Raspberry	164
Açai	185
Rawfood.com Cacao Nibs	621

ORAC Value (umole TE/g)

Brunswick Laboratories Wareham MA USA

To get the best raw chocolate available visit my raw chocolate site at www.yurichocolate.com. You'll be astonished at how delicious raw cacao (chocolate) actually tastes.

Go to www.yurichocolate.com and order yours today!

Sesame Seeds

Sesame seeds are one of the most underrated and poorly understood foods. These seeds are small yet pack a powerful punch full of beneficial nutrients. Most notably, sesame seeds are very high in copper, magnesium, and calcium (#1 food source). Just a quarter-cup of sesame seeds supplies 74% of the daily value (DV) for copper, 31.6% of the DV for magnesium, and 35.1% of the DV for calcium. This rich assortment of minerals translates into many health benefits.

Copper is known for its use in reducing some of the pain and swelling of rheumatoid arthritis. Copper's effectiveness is due to the fact that this trace mineral is important in a number of anti-inflammatory and antioxidant enzyme systems. In addition, copper plays an important role in the activity of *lysyl oxidase*, an enzyme needed for the cross-linking of collagen and elastin - the ground substances that provide structure, strength and elasticity in blood vessels, bones, and joints.

The magnesium inherent in sesame seeds is well known to support vascular and respiratory health. Some of its roles include: preventing airway spasm in asthma, lowering high blood pressure, preventing the trigeminal blood vessel spasm that triggers migraine attacks, and restoring normal sleep patterns in women experiencing unpleasant symptoms associated with menopause.

Everyone knows that calcium is important to the body, but not everyone may know the benefits to be had by consuming sesame seeds! As the #1 source of calcium, sesame seeds protect colon cells from cancer-causing chemicals and help prevent bone loss that can occur as a result of menopause or other conditions such as rheumatoid arthritis. They help prevent migraine headaches in those who suffer from them and reduce PMS symptoms during the luteal phase (the second half) of the menstrual cycle. Sesame seeds even provide the necessary calcium components for muscular contraction.

Sesame seeds are so easy to enjoy. Many of the recipes in this book add sesame seeds not only for their slight taste but for their powerful nutritional properties. Tahini (ground sesame), the base for hummus, is a perfect example. I usually throw a few tablespoons of ground sesame seeds into most of my smoothies to give them an extra boost of alkalizing minerals. To grind sesame seeds into Tahini simply throw the seeds into a coffee grinder and pulse them until they become powder-like and begin to stick together.

Quinoa

Commonly considered a grain, quinoa is actually a relative of leafy green vegetables like spinach and Swiss chard. A recently rediscovered ancient "grain" native to South America, quinoa was once called "the gold of the Incas," because they recognized its value in increasing the stamina of their warriors. Not only is quinoa high in protein at roughly 30% but the protein it supplies is complete, meaning it includes all nine essential amino acids. Not only is quinoa's amino acid profile well balanced, making it a good choice for vegans concerned about adequate protein intake, but it is especially well-endowed with the amino acid lysine, essential for tissue growth and repair.

In addition to protein, quinoa features a host of other health-building nutrients. It is a very good source of manganese and a good source of magnesium, iron, copper, phosphorous, and B vitamins. For this reason, quinoa may be especially valuable for persons with migraine headaches, diabetes and atherosclerosis. Quinoa has powerful antioxidant properties and its fiber and lignan content helps lower the risk for Type II Diabetes, helps prevent gallstone formation, and protects against heart disease.

Because quinoa is a whole food and not subjected to processing, it is not a common allergenic food and is a nice alternative to typical grains such as white rice and wheat breads and pastas. It should be rinsed thoroughly before cooking or sprouting in order to remove the saponin ("soaplike") coating. It is wonderful to use as a base for salads, cereals, and dips like tabouli or hummus.

Nori

Nori is the sea vegetable (aka. Seaweed) used to make sushi. It is a wonderfully nutritious seaweed that can be used as an alternative to bread when making sandwiches or wraps. You can even make your own sushi (see the Healthy Recipe Guide) in no time. Nori comes in dark green sheets and is nearly 50% protein! It is also high in fiber and an extremely valuable source of sea-based minerals including iodine. Iodine is important since it supports the thyroid gland, which is the gland that controls your body's metabolism. Many people with an underactive thyroid can benefit greatly from consuming more sea vegetables.

Nearly 40% of nori's dry weight is minerals. Most people these days are eating mineral-void foods because of depleted soils and the higher cost of mineral-rich organic foods. Sea vegetables like nori, kelp, kombu, wakame, arame, and dulse are great avenues for ensuring adequate mineral intake. Nobel Prize winner Dr. Linus Pauling even said that all diseases can be traced back to a mineral deficiency. So eat more sea vegetables and you'll be off to a great start!

Kale

Kale is a leafy green vegetable that belongs to the Brassica family, a group of cruciferous vegetables that includes cabbage, collards and Brussels sprouts. They have gained recent widespread attention due to their health promoting, sulfur-containing phytonutrients. Kale contains 1300%, 192%, and 88% of the daily value for vitamin K, A, and C, respectively. Vitamin A is a powerful antioxidant well known for lowering the risk of developing cataracts and supporting healthy lung function by protecting the mucous lining of the airways.

Kale is also an important source of iron which helps in the prevention of anemia and the building of strong healthy red blood cells. According to the **USDA Handbook No. 456**, gram for gram, kale has 14 times more iron than red meat! And because vitamin C helps iron absorption, the high levels of vitamin C in kale significantly help the body's ability to assimilate the iron inherent in kale. Just another example of the perfection naturally present in whole foods.

Numerous studies have shown that diets rich in cruciferous vegetables are associated with lower incidence of a variety of cancers including lung, breast, colon, ovarian, and bladder. For instance, in the **Netherlands Cohort Study on Diet and Cancer** in which data was collected on over 100,000 people for more than 6 years, those eating the most vegetables benefited with a 25% lower risk of colorectal cancers. However, those eating the most cruciferous vegetables (ie. kale, broccoli) - only 3 to 5 servings per week - did almost twice as well with a 49% drop in their colorectal cancer risk. [30]

Most notably, kale has been noted for its sulfur-containing phytonutrients. These compounds actually signal your genes to increase the production of enzymes involved in detoxification, the cleansing process through which the body eliminates harmful

---

[30] Voorrips LE, Goldbohm RA, et al. Vegetable and fruit consumption and risks of colon and rectal cancer in a prospective cohort study: The Netherlands Cohort Study on Diet and Cancer. Am J Epidemiol. 2000 Dec 1;152(11):1081-92. PMID:11117618.

compounds. Because of these *organosulfurs*, kale is a liver-friendly food that helps keep the liver in good health.

Look for kale with firm, deeply colored leaves and moist hardy stems. Kale should be displayed in a cool environment since warm temperatures will cause it to wilt and will negatively affect its flavor. The leaves should look fresh and unwilted, free from signs of browning, yellowing and small holes. Choose kale with smaller-sized leaves since these will be tenderer and have a milder flavor than those with larger leaves. Kale is at its peak from the middle of winter through the beginning of spring although it is available all year round.

Kale should be wrapped in a damp paper towel, placed in a plastic bag and stored in the refrigerator crisper. It should not be washed before storing since this may cause it to wilt. Kale can be kept in the refrigerator for several days, although it is best when eaten within one or two days after purchase. The longer it is stored the more bitter its flavor will become.

Maca

This is a powdered supplement that originates from the Peruvian maca root. It contains amino acids, complex carbohydrates, vitamins B, C, and E, and many important minerals such as calcium, phosphorous, zinc, magnesium, and iron. Its many benefits include the balancing of hormones, building muscle, enhancing stamina, and increasing fertility. Most notably is its ability to support the adrenal glands and alleviate stress on the body. For this reason, I highly recommend it for anyone who is stressed and/or has adrenal fatigue.

Maca has a strong, funny taste, almost like a powdered sweet potato. It goes best in smoothies that contain strong flavours.

Flax (seed and oil)

Flaxseeds are included in this list of superfoods for 3 main reasons. First, they are a great source of omega-3 essential fatty acids (more prominent in flaxseed oil). We've already discussed the importance of an omega-3 rich diet. Second, flaxseeds are an incredible source of fiber. Fiber is important because it adds bulk to the stool, lowers cholesterol and the risk of cardiovascular disease, and moderates blood sugar – just to name a few benefits. Third, flax is the highest plant source of lignans - compounds that are increasingly being studied for their potential benefits to both men's and women's health. Flax lignans are being hailed as one of the emerging new health ingredients.

Lignans are phytonutrients found in unrefined grains, legumes, certain vegetables and seeds. Flax is the richest source of lignans, providing 75 – 800 times more lignans than most other plant sources. Lignans have numerous biological properties. They are phytoestrogens, or naturally occurring plant estrogens, that can have a balancing effect on hormones. Lignans also exhibit strong antioxidant activities. They have been studied extensively and research has shown lignans to be beneficial for the health of the bones, the prostate, the breasts, and the heart, while reducing symptoms of menopause and minimizing hair loss, acne, and inflammation.

Flaxseeds have been shown to have similar cholesterol-lowering benefits to statin drugs. In a study involving 40 patients with high cholesterol (greater than 240 mg/dL), daily consumption of 20 grams of ground flaxseed was compared to taking a statin drug. After 60 days, significant reductions were seen in total cholesterol, LDL cholesterol, triglycerides and the ratio of total to HDL cholesterol-in both groups. Those receiving flaxseed did just as well as those given statin drugs![31]

Flaxseeds should be purchased whole and organic. However, because our body's digestive tract cannot break down these tough seeds, it is important to grind them in a coffee grinder before adding them to your foods. Grinding them exposes their precious

---

[31] Mandasescu S, Mocanu V, Dascalita AM, Haliga R, Nestian I, Stitt PA, Luca V. Flaxseed supplementation in hyperlipidemic patients. Rev Med Chir Soc Med Nat Iasi. 2005 Jul-Sep;109(3):502-6. PMID:16607740.

omega-3 oils and other fragile phytonutrients. Once ground they should be consumed immediately or stored in the freezer. Ground flaxseeds are a great addition to cereals, smoothies, and any other dish that requires thickening.

8 Bring in the Reinforcements
4 Essential Supplements

Although the approach in this book is one of natural whole foods, I still believe that most people can benefit from a few essential supplements that are tougher to attain solely through foods. Just remember that these are "supplements" and not "replacements". The purpose of these 4 supplements is to reinforce your already healthy diet.

Probiotics and Prebiotics

Probiotic supplements are simply supplements that contain "friendly" bacteria that you want in the digestive tract in large numbers. Prebiotics [ie. fructo-oligossacharides (FOS), short-chain fatty acids such as butyrate, and inulin] contain the nutrients that these bacteria need to grow and thrive. There are over 400 different types of these friendly bacteria in your colon that serve to complete the digestion of undigested foods, keep pathogenic bacteria and yeasts in check, add bulk to your stool, and produce vitamin K and some of the B vitamins. Until recently, the importance of a healthy and balanced gut flora (bacteria) has been neglected, but thankfully much research has shown its importance not only to the health of your colon, but to your overall health.

Dysbiosis, the imbalance between healthy and unhealthy flora in the colon, is very common in today's society considering how much we abuse our digestive system. If you ever experience intestinal gas, bloating, stomach upset, allergies, or constipation, then you will definitely benefit from probiotics.

The key probiotic bacteria that you want to look for are **bifidobacteria** and **lactobacilli**. Within these categories are many strains but the most helpful for the health of your colon are *Lactobacillus acidophilus, Bifidobacterium bifidum*, and *Streptococcus faecium*. Naturally, yogurts and kefir are good sources of probiotics. However, since I don't endorse the consumption of dairy, the best alternative is to find a high quality probiotic oral supplement. A good probiotic supplement should contain a wide array of bacterial strains, with the 3 mentioned above being the most prominent. Most importantly, ensure that your probiotic supplement contains a suitable number of microorganisms. In general, choose a probiotic supplement that contains anywhere from 6 to 10 billion microorganisms and take the dosage once per day. Good probiotic supplements will also often contain adequate amounts of prebiotics to promote the proliferation of healthy bacteria. In most cases, it's best to take your probiotic on an empty stomach. I find just before bed works best for me.

Incorporating probiotics into your diet will make marked improvements in your digestion, elimination, and overall health. You will notice your bowel movements improve in consistency and regularity, you will help lessen the risk for the development of allergies, and you will dramatically improve the health of your colon and the rest of your body. These friendly bacteria are truly amazing!

Fish Oil

The importance of fish oil has already been discussed in the previous chapter under polyunsaturated fats. However, I thought I'd officially include fish oil in this section because I truly believe that **everyone** can benefit from fish oil in their diet. It has been said that we consume 1/10th of the omega-3s that we need. In fact, our omega-6 to omega-3 is totally out of whack. Most westerners' diets consist of a 10:1 up to 20:1 omega-6 to omega-3 ratio. The problem with this unbalance is that omega-6 fatty acids, depending on the pathway they follow in the body, can be readily converted to inflammatory prostaglandins. Omega-3 fatty acids on the other can only be converted into the highly beneficial anti-inflammatory prostaglandin 1 and 3 molecules. Therefore, choosing a high quality fish oil rich in omega-3 (EPA/DHA) can be highly beneficial to your health.

The scientific literature consistently shows that fish oil is of great benefit to the cardiovascular system, nervous system, and immune system. It helps lessen symptoms of depression, slows the aging process, preserves memory and brain function, is needed for proper cell membrane function, is helpful for diabetes, and may prevent certain cancers and improve treatment outcomes in others.

When choosing a fish oil, look for one that has come from **smaller fish** (sardines, anchovies, krill, mackerel, arctic cod, and herring) as they have less potential for toxic residue buildup. Also, be sure that the oil has been **molecularly distilled** to remove all potential toxins.

Fish oil can be enjoyed by adding it to your smoothies, juices, or straight up. Although the daily recommended intake for omega-3 fatty acids is roughly 2-3 grams, there have been no studies showing that higher dosages harm the body in any way. I usually take 1-2 tbsp of fish oil per day.

Whey Protein

Although *Eating for Energy* is truly about plant-based whole foods, I firmly believe that it is our job to nourish our bodies with the best possible nutrients. In the case of whey protein, which comes from bovine, it just so happens that this is by far the best source of supplemental protein. If you are a physically active individual, constantly stressing your body's muscles and immune system, and feel that supplemental protein is necessary, then whey is probably your best bet. I also recommend the plant-based hemp protein to those who are absolutely strict vegan but please remember that hemp protein is dwarfed by the biological value and overwhelming health-promoting benefits of whey protein. Therefore, it is my duty to present this fantastic protein supplement to you. In fact, as you'll see, it's more than just a protein source. Whether you use it or not is up to you.

Whey is one of two major sources of protein in milk (casein protein being the other). When milk is turned into cheese, the whey protein is filtered out. Whey protein is very easily digested and utilized by the body. Biological Value (BV) is a term you will often see used with regards to protein powders. BV is a measure of the efficiency with which protein can be absorbed and utilized by the body for tissue growth - the higher the value the greater the efficiency. Egg protein is the standard for BV as it was at the top when the scale debuted. Egg protein has a BV of 100. Milk (casein and whey) comes in at around 85, beef proteins around 75. By comparison, the protein in most grains, nuts, beans, and vegetables have a BV of 70-80. Whey protein supplements in the concentrated form have a BV of around 104 whereas whey in an isolated form can have a BV approaching 170!

Whey efficiently builds and repairs muscle tissue, contains all the essential and non-essential amino acids, increases human growth hormone, and lowers cortisol (the stress hormone) production. Whey has also been shown to regulate immune function and is therefore very beneficial to those suffering from compromised immunity or auto-immune conditions such as HIV, lupus, rheumatoid arthritis, and multiple sclerosis. One of the reasons for its immune support is that whey contains microfractions that are natural antiviral, antibacterial, and antifungal agents. Another powerful reason for choosing whey is that it is one of the only protein sources that is alkalizing in the body!

Whey has also been found to protect against some of the toxic effects of chemotheraphy while supporting and protecting non-cancerous cells. It has also been shown to protect against colon and prostate cancer!

When it comes to heart health, whey also has its place by helping reduce cholesterol and blood pressure in hypertensive individuals.

Whey even helps you maintain a healthy weight. Here are 4 ways that whey helps keep you thin:

1. Increases and supports muscle – the more muscle you have the more calories you burn. It's that simple.
2. Balances blood sugar – moderates the glycemic index of ingested carbohydrates preventing them from being converted into fat.
3. Takes more energy to digest and absorb protein than carbohydrates or fat – As a result, you burn more calories eating protein (NOTE: I do not promote low carb, high protein diets!!!)
4. Whey controls appetite – a compound in whey called *glycomacropeptide* acts as a mild appetite suppressant.

If you've ever been to a health food store and noticed the plethora of whey proteins to choose from, you, like most people, must have been quite overwhelmed and confused as to which one to select. With the following information I hope to make your job a lot easier by giving you the essentials of what to look for when selecting a high quality whey protein powder. The 2 main things to look for are that you obtain a whey protein **isolate** that has gone through **cross flow microfiltration**. Here's why...

1. **Choose ISOLATE instead of CONCENTRATE**

   First, whey protein isolate is 90% protein per serving (concentrate is only 80% per serving) and has a BV of about 150 to 170 meaning that it is highly absorbed and utilized in your body. Second, it has NO cholesterol whereas whey concentrate has about 40 mg of cholesterol. Third, isolate has a lower percent of fat per serving and is only 0.1 - 0.3% lactose compared to 2 - 5% lactose in concentrate form. This can be an important consideration for those who are sensitive to lactose.

2. **Look for whey that has undergone CROSS FLOW MICROFILTRATION (CFM)**

   Cross Flow Microfiltration is a natural, non-chemical process to isolate a pure quality protein product. Cross Flow Microfiltration can produce better quality whey protein than Ion-Exchange (another common method used). That is because the chemicals used in Ion-Exchange denature some proteins and amino acids. As a result, most of whey's therapeutic properties are lost when processed through Ion-Exchange. Therefore, in order to retain whey's amazing health benefits and fully un-denatured proteins choose CFM.

Glutamine

Glutamine is the most abundant amino acid in the body. In fact, it could almost be the king of amino acids due to its numerous benefits. Glutamine is converted to glucose when more glucose is required by the body as an energy source. Glutamine also serves as a source of fuel for cells lining the intestines. Without it, these cells waste away. It is also used by white blood cells and is important for immune function.

Few healthy people are glutamine deficient, in part because the body makes its own. During fasting, starvation, cirrhosis, critical illnesses, and weight loss associated with AIDS and cancer, however, deficiencies often develop.

I recommend glutamine for 2 reasons:

First, it is the most effective nutritional agent for repairing the intestinal lining. This is critically important as a damaged gut (leaky gut) is at the root of many problems in the body. By using glutamine to help repair the cells of the intestinal lining, you help your digestive function and reduce the possibility for allergy development. Glutamine is clearly the preferred fuel source of the cells (enterocytes) of the small intestine, even more so than glucose! Hospitals are even adding glutamine to tube-fed and intravenous formulas because of its amazing benefits to the intestinal lining.

Second, glutamine is one of the most amazing supplements for promoting muscle tissue repair and growth and for supporting the immune system. For those looking to develop strong and lean muscle or improve their athletic performance glutamine can be of tremendous benefit. Intense exercise can be taxing on the athlete's immune system. Glutamine's immune supporting ability has been well documented in preventing injuries, infections, and colds in intense exercising athletes.

Indeed, a study performed in 1996 by L. M. Castell and his team of researchers looked at the incidence of infections in athletes undertaking prolonged strenuous exercise based on evidence that cells in the immune system are less able to mount a defense against infection after exercise. The researchers monitored levels of infection in 200 runners and rowers and found that levels of infection were highest in those running the full marathon distance or further. They took blood samples from middle distance and marathon runners for the measurement of plasma glutamine and found that a 5g dose of glutamine after strenuous exercise increased plasma glutamine levels markedly with levels returning to near normal about 2 hours after ingestion. Athletes taking part in the study also reported less incidence of infection within 7 days of intense, exhaustive and prolonged exercise after taking glutamine. Indeed, 80% of those in the group ingesting glutamine reported no infections or colds compared to only 48% in the control group drinking a placebo maltodextrin (carbohydrate) drink, a staggering 32% difference. The study concluded that the provision of a glutamine supplement after exercise and then again 2 hours later decreased the risk of infection in athletes completing exhaustive and prolonged exercise. Sounds like the equivalent of discovering the Holy Grail, for distance runners![32]

Glutamine also helps maintain cell volume and hydration, speeding up wound and damaged tissue healing. Glutamine's healing powers have even stretched so far as to assist in peptic ulcer repair!

Raw cabbage juice is an excellent source of glutamine. Otherwise, choosing an L-glutamine powder supplement is most convenient. There are no known side effects of high levels of glutamine intake but taking excessive amounts can lead to stomach upsets. It's safest to follow the instructions on whichever glutamine supplement you purchase. Usually 2 to 5 grams per day is suitable for most active individuals.

[32] LM Castell, EA Newsholme, JR Poortmans (1996). Does glutamine have a role in reducing infections in athletes? European Journal of Applied Physiology. 73 (5): 488-490.

9 Making the Transition

Ok, so now that you've got all this information, how do you go about putting these considerations into practice? Well, I know that it can be intimidating at first but don't worry! As with anything else you adopt into your life, it does take some getting used to. However, as your body begins to cleanse from the years of toxic buildup and less than optimal eating habits, it will soon vibrate with the energy that you crave!

To help you get started, I've broken this section of the book into a few categories of checklist-type recommendations to help you transition from the old you to the new you! This section will cover several topics and frequently asked questions such as:

1. General transition guidelines

2. Eating healthy on the run – restaurants, traveling, and at work

3. Kitchen Essentials - What you need in your kitchen to get started

4. The 10 Success Habits

General Transition Guidelines

1. **Take control of your thoughts**. What you think about, you bring about. Think about yourself as you could be rather than as you currently are. Your potential is endless and you can have the health, radiance, and energy you deserve. Keep focused on the outcome – your end result. This is the key to achieving any goal you set for yourself.

2. **Be patient and have faith**. Rome wasn't built in a day and neither were you. To transform how you look and feel takes time. Depending on how committed you are to transformation, you will see results sooner or later. I think you will be astonished as to how quickly the body can be transformed! Whichever the case may be for you, have faith you are doing your body good and that the healing powers of natural whole living foods will do their job.

3. **Surround yourself with supportive people.** Negative people who tell you that you are crazy or that what you're doing won't work are poisonous to your progress and health. These types of people are simply projecting onto you what they think and feel about themselves. Maybe they are the ones who are crazy! They would be unable to do what you are doing! As Eleanor Roosevelt once said, *"What other people think of me is none of my business!"* So, spend more time with people who are positive and who will encourage and support you!

4. **Transition smoothly away from a meat-based diet**. I would advise to first let go of red meat, then pork, then chicken, and then fish. You can replace meat with avocados, young coconuts, olives, nuts, and seeds. As you move away from meat and into more of a vegetarian diet you will feel happier, less hostile or aggressive, and your energy will skyrocket.

5. **Likewise, transition smoothly away from dairy foods.** Dairy has no place in your diet. First, let go of milk, then cheese. If you simply cannot live without dairy, then move to raw organic milk or cheese. Replacing dairy foods with green leafy vegetables and sesame seeds for calcium and avocados, young coconuts, olives, nuts/seeds for their excellent plant-based fat content. Just imagine a world without mucus and congestion – it can be yours!

6. **Transition away from cooked starches such as wheat and other glutenous grains.** Breads, cereals, and pastas are all cooked grain products that are best minimized and/or avoided. Wheat is one of the top allergenic foods in our society since it is way too abundant and over-processed. Opt for non-glutenous grains such as quinoa, amaranth, millet, buckwheat, and brown rice. These are much healthier for you and can be sprouted or cooked (if you must!). Instead of bread, choose rice cakes. Instead of white pasta, choose rice pasta (which is still cooked but better) or a raw veggie pasta (as described in the Healthy Recipe Guide)

7. **Continue eating a large percentage of raw plant foods** throughout your transition. Using the recipes in this book will greatly assist you in doing so.

8. Depending on how toxic your body is as you begin to transition to plant-based raw foods **you may begin to experience some symptoms of detoxification. That's OK!** These symptoms may include headaches, skin outbreaks, and the reappearance of past conditions – just to name a few. I don't mean to scare you but it's important to realize that if your body is fairly toxic to begin with it will expel these toxins from the inside out. You may experience a "healing crisis" whereby physical and emotional issues from your past that have been buried deep inside, may begin to surface. This is part of the process and will surely pass. Be sure to drink plenty of water to facilitate the elimination of waste from your body and speed up the detoxification process. Detoxifying the body is the first essential stage in healing it. Transition at your own pace but continue to move

forward. To be successful in anything, you must be willing to step outside of your comfort zone.

9. **Eat wild, home grown or local organic foods whenever possible**. Organic food is grown without pesticides and other dangerous chemicals. Over time, consuming large quantities of non-organic foods can dramatically overload your body's immune system as such chemicals can exceed your body's toxic load. Although organic foods are more expensive do your best to choose them especially when buying berries, dates, carrots, pears, cabbage, lemons, grapes, sweet potatoes, peaches, and cherries. These foods are typically sprayed with the greatest amount of pesticides. Buying locally grown is another important element to your health and to the health of the planet. Choosing locally grown foods ensures that you eat seasonally (which is really the best for your body), reduces the energy expenditure of long distance transportation, and supports local farmers. The more you support local organic farmers, the more you support sustainable agriculture and the preservation of our precious soils.

10. **Eat more sweet fruit and/or seeds if you are active**. You will need the sugars and healthy fats. Eat more green leafy vegetables and/or non-sweet fruit if you are more sedentary. But I know that you fall into the active category, right!?

11. **Be aware that certain cooked-food cravings present themselves when you are tired, depressed, and lazy**. Therefore, drink a glass of water to curb your appetite until you get your head around making a healthy food choice. Eat a piece of fruit to tide you over! Do something that makes you feel good, happy, and energized. Don't give in to the little voice in your head that's craving the junk. Take a nap if you need to. Just do your best not to give in. I know it's tough! My downfall is pizza – but I've made leaps and bounds and I know you can too! Cravings are always temporary and usually related to the very foods to which you are sensitive or allergic. Do your best to avoid them and you will reap the benefits physically, mentally, and emotionally.

12. **Eat when you are hungry and choose foods that agree with you.** Don't force things down, especially if you don't like them!

13. **Be sure to exercise each day, in some way, shape or form.** By exercising you will unconsciously start to make better food choices and adopt healthier lifestyle practices.

14. **If you are interested in eating a 100% raw diet, I recommend initially experimenting with it on a small scale.** First go 100% raw for a day. Then extend it to a couple of days, then to a week, or a month. Set in advance a specific date and mark each successful raw day in your calendar. Understand that after you go 100% raw for about 6 months straight, your body will not readily accommodate a return to cooked foods because you will be too cleansed, sensitized, and purified for your body to handle other foods.

15. **Educate yourself.** Saturate your mind with knowledge, information, and strategies to help you in your journey to greatness! Seek out other raw food books, attend raw food cooking classes, or join a group of raw food enthusiasts.

Healthy Eating on the Run

Let's face it – no one has time for anything anymore! The majority of us live in a fast paced world where convenience is king. Processed foods, although convenient and time efficient, will do your body NO good, robbing you of energy rather than providing it. Most of them are loaded with preservatives, sodium, and chemicals which most people cannot even pronounce. It's important to do your best and make the healthiest possible food choices in any given situation. All I ask is that you do the best you can with the knowledge and resources you have. After all, the choice is yours.

Eating in Restaurants

Who doesn't like going out to eat? Eating out with friends, family, or your loved one is what life's about (ok, maybe not – I just got a little excited)! Most cultural traditions revolve around food and socializing. I think it's great and absolutely support it. However, when you are faced with going out for dinner, healthy dishes (let alone raw plant-based ones) aren't necessarily readily available. So here are some recommendations to help you make the most of your dinners out while still enjoying the experience.

1. **Keep it simple.** Choose dishes that are fresh and use simple ingredients. Eating heavy dishes with sauces from unknown sources is a disaster waiting to happen.

2. **Try vegetarian options when possible.** Instead of steak, chicken, or fish try a veggie-based dish. Also notice how light and comfortable you will feel afterwards. It's nicer than the feeling of being excessively full and ready for bed.

3. **Choose a salad instead of French fries or baked potato.** Ask for dressing on the side.

4. **Go for lighter meals.** Avoid heavy, fatty, and deep fried dishes.

5. **Start your meal with a glass of lukewarm lemon water** before eating. This will assist digestion.

6. **Instead of a main course, try sharing several appetizers** with your dinner guests. This is a great way to try different foods that are usually a lot lighter and still satisfying. However, I'm not referring to wings, nachos, cheese bread, etc...

7. **Order vegetables** with anything that you order.

8. **If you are going to drink with your meal, enjoy a glass of red wine.** Red wine is abundant in live enzymes that actually assist in digestion. However, let's keep it reasonable. One glass (not 1 bottle!) is more than enough.

9. **Carry digestive enzymes (supplements) with you to aid digestion.** Take a few capsules before, during, and/or after the meal as needed. Note that carrying exogenous enzymes does not give you an excuse to eat whatever you want!

10. **Avoid eating dessert (and fruit) right after your meal.** If you must have something sweet give your body some time to process whatever food it is dealing with before the sweet onslaught. Eating sugary foods on a full stomach leads to excessive fullness, abdominal discomfort, and gas as the sugar begins to ferment on top of undigested food in your stomach. Listen to your body – it will know when it's ready!

Eating While Traveling

Have you ever come across an airline that serves healthy snacks (or meals for that matter)? Have you ever pulled into a service station off the highway to enjoy a glorious vegetable-based meal? If you answered yes to either one of these questions, then please contact me to let me know about your discovery! There are virtually no healthy snacks or on-the-go meals that can be purchased in an airport, on an airplane, or while driving along the highway. So what can you do to avoid falling asleep at the wheel after a stop-over meal or minimize your chances of feeling like death after airplane foods? Well, here is a list of simple tips to help you get great and convenient nutrition while traveling. The key to healthy eating on the run is planning ahead.

1. **Pack several small snacks.** Fill a Ziploc bag with some nuts, seeds, chopped up apple, or any other combination you enjoy. My personal snack mix of choice is a combination of raw cacao nibs, goji berries, pumpkin seeds, and almonds/walnuts. Amazing nutrition and pure energy! I once played a soccer game after having that mix as my pre-game meal (not necessarily recommended for optimal performance, but boy was I flying!)

2. **Have a water bottle with you at all times.** This is especially important if you're flying, as the dry stale air in the cabin dries your body right out. Try to avoid coffee since it has a diuretic effect and will promote quicker dehydration.

3. **Prepare some transportable meals ahead of time.** You can make a salad to take with you and keep the dressing in a separate container. You can even make a seaweed wrap, keep it in Tupperware, and take it with you. How about freshly made dips like hummus along with some cut up vegetables? You can take some of the energy bars and puddings (described in the Nutrition for Athlete's section). The choices are endless. The key is to be prepared.

4. If traveling to a foreign country (especially to Mexico or Europe), **take advantage of the locally grown produce.**

5. **If you are in a less developed country with a questionable water supply, boil your water to kill any parasites and bacteria**, then recharge it by placing sea salt, fresh lemon juice, MSM powder, and large quartz crystals (if available) in the water before drinking it.

Eating at Work

If you work for yourself and are home-based then you obviously have the luxury of preparing healthy meals at home. But what happens if your stuck in a corporate office for most the day? What do you do for food? Do you hop down to the nearest food court and grab the nastiest of the food court food? Sometimes it may seem as if there's little to no choice. Believe me I know! I recently conducted a little experiment in downtown Toronto. I looked at a very busy intersection in the city and said to myself "Let's see how many healthy food options I can find within a 2 km radius of this intersection!" To my disbelief, I only found 3. However, the fast food restaurants, pizza joints, bagel stops, and hot dog vendors were more abundant than I could keep track of. There is obviously a very serious problem with this scenario. I'm sure your city is the same.

Considering there are few healthy on-the-go options for the worker who is not home-based, the key to healthy eating lies in your ability to plan and prepare your meals ahead of time. The recipes later in this book are great examples of amazingly nutritious and delicious meals that take no more than 10 minutes to make. Whether you're preparing to take them to work or enjoying them when you get home, they are truly convenient healthy options for most people. But for now here are some quick and easy tips to help you eat healthier at work.

1. **Follow tips 1-3 from the Eating While Traveling section** above. The same rules apply.

2. **Avoid sodas and high sugar snack foods that are common in most workplaces.** Choose water and/or herbal teas as your fluid and fresh vegetables, fruit, and nuts and seeds as your snack.

3. **Keep some food at work.** If a refrigerator is available, store some of your healthier foods. If not, you can keep dried foods (ie. nuts, seeds, dried fruit) in your office for convenience.

4. **Locate and frequent (if needed) local produce markets and/or healthy food restaurants that are close to your work.** Knowing where to get healthy foods in tight situations can be a life saver.

5. **Appoint a group of colleagues to be accountable to.** Tell them to ensure that you stay on track. Better yet, get them to join you in your quest for a healthier, more energetic life!

Kitchen Essentials – What You Need to Get Started

Because adopting more of a raw vegetarian diet requires no heating or cooking of foods, most conventional appliances are not even necessary. Stove tops, ovens, microwaves, toasters, and barbecues are not required to enjoy the recipes in this book. However, having these appliances (except for the microwave) is always nice to have around for the rare cooked food occasion.

What follows is a list of utensils and small appliances to get your kitchen ready for the Eating for Energy lifestyle.

Utensils

- Chef's knife – top quality is recommended here.
- Potato peeler
- Spiralizer
- Spatula
- Basic forks, knives, and spoons
- Cheese grater (used for garlic and ginger)
- Tupperware or glassware storage containers
- Ziploc freezer bags

Small Appliances

- Food processor
- High speed blender or Vita-Mix
- Citrus juicer
- Juicer or juice extractor
- Refrigerator/Freezer
- Coffee grinder

The 10 Success Habits

Success Habit 1: Eat one big green salad every day

Success Habit 2: Drink one fresh-pressed green juice or green smoothie every day

Success Habit 3: Balance your meals with carbohydrates, fiber, healthy fats, amino acids and plenty of colour. Practice proper food combining when possible.

Success Habit 4: Drink a glass of lemon water first thing each morning and a half hour before meals.

Success Habit 5: Eat every 2-3 hours (but not if you're not hungry)

Success Habit 6: Drink water throughout the day (1/2 your body weight (lbs) in ounces)

Success Habit 7: Eat meat (and dairy) no more than 2 times per week – Choose soaked/sprouted grains/legumes/nuts/seeds and green leafy vegetables instead.

Success Habit 8: Eat 80% whole living foods (raw)

Success Habit 9: Avoid NON-FOODS (ie. refined sugars, coffee, processed/packaged foods, etc...) as best as possible.

Success Habit 10: Ensure variety and rotation in your meals.

10 pH Balance and Allergies

There are many sources with differing classification for foods along the acid-alkaline (pH balance) forming spectrum. As such, it can be quite confusing for someone to get a definitive and consistent answer for which foods are acid-forming and which are alkalizing. Acid-forming foods are those which leave an acid residue once metabolized by the body. An acid is a chemical compound that, once dissolved in water, lowers the pH of a solution below 7.0. On the other hand, alkaline-forming foods are those which leave an alkaline residue once metabolized by the body. An alkaline substance (or base) is one that has a free pair of electrons to bind a hydrogen ion or make a substance less acidic. Ok, now that you are absolutely lost lets fast-forward to what this means for foods and their effect on your body.

The most accurate way of measuring a food's acid or alkaline forming capacity is by referring to its PRAL (potential renal acid load). PRAL is measured by taking a food's protein and phosphorus content (acid forming) and then subtracting from that the food's content of magnesium, potassium, and calcium (alkaline minerals). The end result is a fairly accurate picture of any given food's effect on the body, from a pH perspective. Please keep in mind that I'm referring to the pH effect or "ash" that a given food creates in the body after it has been metabolized, not before it has been ingested. For instance, citrus fruits are acidic outside of the body but are highly alkaline once metabolized.

What follows is a list of various foods according to their classification as being acid or alkaline-forming in the body.

Typical North American Diet

Foods	Slightly-Alkaline Forming	Neutral	Acid-Forming	Highly Acid-Forming
				Commercial breakfast cereal
				Pasta
				Refined wheat flour
Grains				White Rice
				Bagels, Bread
Meat			Cold-Water Fish	Beef
			Venison	Pork
			Wild Game	Poultry
				Shellfish
Dairy			Milk (raw, unprocessed)	Butter
				Cheese (all)
				Cream
				Milk (pasteurized)
Sugars/Sweeteners				Sugar (all types)
				Artificial Sweeteners

Miscellaneous	Synthetic multivitamins	Candy
		Coffee
		Soft Drinks
		Soy/Whey protein
		Margarine

Eating For Energy Foods

Foods	Highly-Alkaline Forming	Alkaline-Forming	Neutral	Slightly Acid-Forming
Grains				Brown rice
Non-Gluten Grains		Quinoa		
				Millet
				Amaranth
		Buckwheat		
Legumes				Black beans
				Black-eyed peas
				Chickpeas
				Lentils
Seeds		Sesame	Flax	Pumpkin
			Hemp	Sunflower
Nuts			Macadamia	Almonds
		Coconut	Walnuts	
Fruit	ALL			
Vegetables	ALL			

Source: USDA database (rev. 18).

As you can easily tell, the difference between the Standard American Diet (SAD) or Western Diet and that of *Eating for Energy* is quite different. The typical SAD is very acid forming and thus is highly correlated with illness, lethargy, weight gain, poor athletic performance, and a shortened lifespan. Conversely, *Eating for Energy* foods are highly alkalizing and provide your body with the nutrients and pH balance it requires. It has been said that for optimal health, our diet should be 80% alkaline and only 20% acidic. However, after looking at these tables we can see that quite the reverse holds true for the majority of people living in Westernized countries.

The amusing part, though, is that the leading governmental authorities actually encourage us to eat more closely to that of which is being described in *Eating for Energy*.

Fewer Allergies Means Better Health

I must say that I'm not a believer of fad diets and I don't believe that there is ever one diet that is suitable for all people all the time. Having said that, humans are humans. Although we all have our own biochemical makeup, we typically respond well to foods that are healthy for us, while presenting symptoms of ill health when consuming foods artificial in nature.

Consider the startling example of the Hunza people who live in the Himalayas. Often living well into their hundreds, the Hunza were well known for remaining active and eating an alkalizing diet consisting mainly of raw fruits and vegetables and sun-baked breads. The diseases of the Western world were unknown to these people. However, when westerners began building railroads into the mountainous region they introduced processed foods to these formerly untouched people. Within one year, the first case of cancer was detected among the Hunza people. Today these people have many of the same diseases that are plaguing the Western world, and their lifespan has decreased dramatically.

The food philosophy presented in this book is one that is healthy, alkalizing, nourishing, and empowers your body. Furthermore it is hypoallergenic. This means that the common food allergens – dairy, wheat, soy, peanuts, corn, yeast, eggs, alcohol – as well as pesticides and other chemicals do not have a place in this approach.

The benefit of following a hypoallergenic way of eating is that fewer burdens are placed on your digestive and immune systems, so there is less likelihood that food intolerances and/or food allergies will be present. Allergies and food intolerances are a serious issue. Do not take them lightly. Dr. Bateson-Koch even entitled her book **Allergies – Disease in Disguise**! It's a very good book and I would highly recommend reading it.

Although several foods and recipes are recommended in this book, if you find your body doesn't agree with any particular one then that is a sign you probably shouldn't be eating those foods. For instance, my girlfriend will often experience itchy skin and eczema when she eats dates. These symptoms do not appear if those dates are organic.

Two hallmark symptoms of food allergies/sensitivities are fatigue and headaches. If you experience them after your meals use that as feedback to not continue eating those foods! However, food allergies/sensitivities can manifest themselves in many different ways. Other signs and symptoms of food allergies/sensitivities include frequent night urination, mucus production, runny or stuffy nose, rapid heart rate (after eating allergenic food), and many others.

You can develop an allergy to any food that is present in the body far too often. Here are 2 main ways the body can develop food allergies:

1. **Eating Large Quantities of a Particular Food and Eating That Food Far Too Frequently (several times a day or on consecutive days)**
   This is especially true with cooked foods. The reason is that when you overly consume a given food, your body eventually runs out of the enzyme necessary to digest that food. For instance, if you eat eggs every single day, over time you're likely to deplete your body's specific enzymes for digesting eggs and your body will

become intolerant to them. This occurs to a much lesser extent with living foods since these foods contain enzymes that assist in their own digestion.

2. **Food Sits in Your Digestive Tract Far Too Long**
   If foods are not being digested properly and not moving efficiently through your intestines, these foods will literally stick to the intestinal walls where they will give off toxins, irritate the mucosal lining, feed bad bacteria, and trigger immune responses. Over time, this food can build up and become impacted onto the walls of the intestines creating a "mucoid plaque". If this develops (and in fact it does for the majority of people in western countries) it reduces the lumen (the center of the intestines) and prevents nutrients from being absorbed and assimilated into your body. Think about it – how can your body absorb nutrients if the intestines are coated with layers of impacted food? Nutrients can't get through! You will most likely notice loose stools since your body is trying to rid itself of the "foreign invaders" that are upsetting your digestive system.

This is just another reason to ensure that your bowel movements are solid, smooth in passing, and are frequent throughout the day. You should be passing a bowel movement at least twice a day and ideally after every meal. Eating whole living foods that don't upset your body and drinking plenty of water throughout the day will help you in this department.

Following **Success Habit #10 – Ensuring variety and rotation in your meals** – will help lessen the possibility of developing sensitivities to the foods you enjoy. By following the 12-Week Meal Plan later in this book, you'll notice how meals and foods are rotated so that the same food/meal isn't consumed on consecutive days.

11 The 5 Essential Pillars

In order to have more energy, achieve your ideal weight, be fit and strong, live a long and healthy life free of disease there are 5 essential pillars you must work toward incorporating into your daily life.

1. Alkalize your body
2. Nourish your body with enzyme-rich, living, plant-based whole foods
3. Ameliorate digestion and absorption
4. Reduce stress (emotional, physical, chemical, etc...)
5. Exercise on a regular basis

There is obviously a bit of overlap between elements 1 and 2 but I wanted to separate them because they each deserve special attention.

1. Alkalize Your Body

We have already spent a great deal of time learning why you need to alkalize your body. This section will focus on empowering you with immediate action steps you can take to start doing so immediately.

1. **Eat More Green Vegetables (and all fruits and vegetables for that matter)**

   There's a reason these form the top of the *Eating for Energy* Food Spectrum. Green vegetables are your greatest source of alkalinity due the alkalizing minerals that they provide and the high electrical energy (from the sun) that they transfer to our blood. Remember to get plenty of servings from the RAINBOW COLOURS group of fruits and vegetables. All of these plant-derived foods are terrifically alkalizing and provide a tremendous amount of nutrients, anti-oxidants, flavonoids, and much more to your body. Within any given meal ensure that you have a beautiful array of colours.

2. **Start Your Day with Lemon Water**

   Upon waking, squeeze the juice of ¼ to ½ lemon into a glass (350 ml) of luke warm water. Be sure to use an actual lemon and not lemon juice from concentrate. Lemon has an amazing alkalizing effect on your body and serves to gently cleanse the liver, stimulating gall bladder function and the gastric activity of your stomach. If you don't feel hungry in the morning then this lemon water combo will help get your digestive system started. However, listen to your body. If you're not hungry, don't force food down.

3. **Reduce and/or Eliminate Coffee and Refined Sugars from Your Diet**

   Coffee is by far one of the world's most popular and loved beverages. According to Wirthlin Worldwide (a market research company), North Americans consume on average 1.8 cups of coffee per day. Compare this to our water consumption. It is recommended to consume on average eight to ten 8 oz glasses of "living water" (ie. mineral rich, slightly alkaline, and energy producing within the body) each day.

However, scary statistics reveal that 20% of North Americans drink no water at all while only 42% of us consume a mere 2 glasses or fewer.

Although coffee beans in their original whole state have potent antioxidant properties, once they've been processed and roasted they no longer provide much value to your body. So, before ordering your next "mocha latte frappawhatever" remember the following facts about coffee:

- Coffee intensifies stress, causing an average 40% increase in adrenaline. This results in increased blood pressure, heart rate, perspiration, nervousness, and irritability.
- Coffee increases the secretion of stomach acid by 400%, contributing to gastritis and peptic ulcers.
- According to the British Medical Journal **Lancet,** coffee drinkers have a 50% higher risk of heart attack
- Coffee causes a significant loss of nutrients, especially alkalizing minerals such as magnesium, potassium, calcium, zinc, and B vitamins.
- Coffee is a major source of cadmium, a heavy metal that has been linked to cancer and immune suppression.

If you're a woman, please consider the following even scarier facts:

- Caffeine is linked to ovarian cancer, bladder, and kidney cancers.
- According to the **Journal of the American Medical Association**, coffee increases the risk of miscarriage and can double the rate with just 1 cup (160 mg caffeine) per day!
- Coffee reduces fertility. More than 1 cup per day makes a woman half as likely to conceive (**American Journal of Epidemiology**)!

Please remember that this is by no means an exhaustive list of coffee's effects on the body. Also consider that for each cup (100 mg caffeine) of coffee you should be throwing back 3 cups of purified living water to make up for coffee's diuretic effect. Aside from all these effects, it is vitally important to remember that coffee is acid-forming in the body, and more so if taken with sugar and milk.

For many people, simply reducing coffee from twice a day to once a day is an amazing accomplishment. Right off the bat, that's a 50% decrease. Julie, my tax specialist client who I mentioned in the beginning of the book, would easily drink 3-4 cups of coffee per day. For her this seemed normal. We eventually got her down to 1 cup every few days and she feels absolutely phenomenal!

With her previous coffee consumption, what Julie failed to realize was the evident connection between her caffeine intake and subsequent hypoglycemic states (or low blood sugar). Caffeine is a stimulant (as are refined sugars) and; therefore, triggers the adrenal glands to secrete adrenaline into the blood stream. Once adrenaline has been released into the blood stream it has a catabolic effect and signals the breakdown of glycogen into glucose for the blood. With a sudden rise in blood glucose, insulin is then released to moderate blood sugar levels by taking this glucose and storing it back into the muscle and liver cells. A subsequent drop in blood sugar is then experienced. This initiates a vicious cycle that leads to sugar cravings or more coffee to "fix" the blood sugar imbalance.

In most cases, people will opt for quick fixes like pastries, chocolate bars, coffee, colas, and other sweets to get their blood sugar back up. But because refined sugars are so quickly metabolized, they too spike blood sugar and the entire sequence repeats itself. Eventually, your body's insulin can no longer do its job because the cells have simply become "immune" to its effect. When your body no longer accepts insulin's action, blood sugar remains elevated leading to the development of type II diabetes!

In sum, consumption of acid-forming caffeine (coffee) and refined sugars wreak havoc on your blood sugar levels. If left unchanged, this diet of coffee and sugar will cause your body to become resistant to insulin, which will eventually lead to diabetes. Low blood sugar (hypoglycemia) is an early warning sign for the development of Type II Diabetes. But you can change that!

4. Reduce (and hopefully eliminate...eventually) Consumption of Animal Products

As alluded to earlier, animal products (meat, dairy, eggs, etc...) are highly acid-forming in the body. They are also very difficult for most people to digest properly. Simply reducing how much and how often you eat these "flesh" foods will make a big difference – and your body will thank you. Animal foods are also highly inflammatory in the body due to their significant levels of arachidonic acid. With excess animal consumption come higher levels of inflammation in the body. As the body tries to protect itself from this inflammation it secretes greater amounts of mucus. I have personally seen many "meat-eating" clients dramatically reduce mucus overload in their bodies simply by reducing and eliminating the consumption of animal products.

More importantly, for people who suffer from inflammatory conditions including (but not limited to): osteoarthritis, chronic pulmonary obstructive disease, asthma, colitis, crohn's, pelvic inflammatory disease, eczema, and psoriasis, getting rid of animal products is a must. Inflammation is common to all disease. Less animal consumption means less arachidonic acid, which leads to less inflammation. The only exception to this rule is the occasional consumption of cold water fish which has anti-inflammatory benefits due to its high concentration of omega-3 fatty acids.

If you're concerned about protein intake then just remember that the biggest, strongest, and longest living animals are all vegetarian. The elephant, gorilla, and giraffe are all great animals who subsist on leaves and/or fruit.

Bill Pearl, who won 4 Mr. Universe body-building titles, was completely vegetarian! After having been a huge meat eater for most of his life, Bill had had some blood work done after which his doctor said that his uric acid, blood pressure, and triglycerides were so high that he was a prime candidate for a heart attack! He was advised to remove red meat from his diet and so he did. He describes his experiences with the conversion to vegetarianism.

"With each succeeding year on the diet (lacto-ovo vegetarian), I've felt better. I'm more healthy, I can train with more energy, and I'm not as much of a "hard guy" as I used to be. I've become more concerned with my fellow man and the other inhabitants I share the planet with. ...I have now been vegetarian for almost 20 years. We have no fish, fowl, or red meat in our diet. Yet I can still carry the same amount of muscle as I did in winning my four Mr. Universe titles. People can't believe it. They think that to have big muscles you have to eat meat - it's a persistent and recurring myth. But take it from me, there's nothing magic about eating meat that's going to make you a champion bodybuilder. Anything you can find in a piece of meat, you can find in other foods as well."[33]

Well put Bill.

Even body-builder extraordinaire Arnold Schwarzenegger once said,

"Bill Pearl never talked me into becoming a vegetarian, but he did convince me that a vegetarian could become a champion bodybuilder."

Although Bill Pearl was not a strict raw-foodist, his example clearly demonstrates the power of a whole food plant-based diet. I can only imagine what success he would have achieved had he consumed more raw plant foods.

Following the Eating for Energy philosophy you can easily get enough high quality protein through plant-based sources such as spouted lentils and chic peas, hemp, spirulina, green leafy vegetables, and nuts and seeds. If you feel you need additional protein because of high physical demands then I would recommend supplementing with a whole food hemp protein supplement or a high quality whey protein.

---

[33] Interview with Dennis Weis. Body Building.com.

By consuming too many saturated fat-containing animal products (ie. red meat), and even leaner meats (chicken and fish), you force your stomach and digestive tract to work overtime in order to fully break down heavy proteins into their amino acid building blocks.

Ultimately, your body uses amino acids to build its tissues so why not give your body what it requires right from the start? Plant-based protein sources are much easier to digest since they come in smaller peptide chains and/or individual amino acids. Therefore, your body doesn't have to waste as much energy breaking them down. This is also very helpful for people who have an underactive stomach (like me and about 80% of the population).

By following these 4 steps to alkalize your body, you'll be on your way to a new you – a new life – a new energy!

2. Nourish Your Body with Enzyme-Rich, Living, Plant-Based Whole Foods

Providing your body with living whole foods cannot be underestimated. This is the essence of the *Eating for Energy* nutritional philosophy. However, since most people (including myself) find it difficult to eat 100% raw, I would encourage the following:

1. Eat At Least 80% of Your Foods in Their Whole Living State (Raw)

Slowly but surely begin to incorporate more living whole foods into your diet. Even if everything else stays the same, this alone will make a drastic improvement in your energy, metabolic function, and overall health. By providing your body with the "food enzymes" inherent in living foods you allow your body to conserve its limited store of digestive enzymes while spending more of its energy on circulating its vital "metabolic enzymes" to assist in all other bodily functions.

Remember, cooked food is dead! It's no wonder that so many people walk around like zombies. You are what you eat! Did it ever occur to you that humans are the only species (out of over 2 million) on the planet that eat cooked foods?! Don't you think all living creatures would have adopted cooked foods if they thought it vital to their survival? Well, obviously that hasn't happened. Why then are we so we hung up on cooked foods that deplete and inflame our bodies? I will admit that it is not easy to completely override years of cooked food conditioning but when you begin to experience the difference raw living foods have on your life, you'll have a much easier time. From my experience and the experience of many others the difference is like day and night! It is so profound that attempting to describe it in words cannot even come close to doing it justice. As such, I highly encourage you to start consuming more foods in their living state and reducing your consumption of dead, lifeless, cooked foods!

Heating/cooking alters the structure of protein molecules, making them more difficult to digest which can promote the development of food allergies. For instance, it's generally easier to digest a soft-boiled egg compared to a hard boiled egg. The longer a protein molecule is subjected to high temperatures, the more it becomes denatured and the more difficult it becomes to digest. Remember, your body is best suited to digest whole foods that have not been ravaged by modern technology.

Start by eating at least 80% of your foods in their raw living state. Ideally, it would be great to reach 100% raw food intake but I will admit that this can be challenging especially if you live in colder climates. However, because I recognize the importance of moderation, balance, and sustainability in one's diet, I would rather you listen to your body and satisfy what it needs. But do differentiate between the need for "cravings" such as refined sugars and your body's "calling" for specific nutrient intake. For example, many people crave chocolate not so much for the quick sugar fix but instead because of its high content of magnesium – a mineral in which most are deficient.

Let's assume that you have on average 4 meals/feedings per day. That would amount to 28 meals in one week. Now, let's be conservative and assume that 80% of your diet will be raw foods, meaning that 20% can be cooked or leisure foods. So of the 28 weekly meals, roughly 22 of them should be raw with the other 6 in whatever shape or form you like. This will be easier to adhere to by following the 12-Week Meal Plan later in the book.

As your body begins to transform and your taste buds adjust to this healthier way of eating, you will no longer crave "conventional foods" as you once did. In fact, when you notice the energy draining effect they have on your cleansed body you will no longer even desire them. This is a process but it's absolutely worth every minute of it. If you're serious about improving your health, losing weight, improving performance in all areas of your life, living longer (and in optimal health), and want the best life ever, then this process must be undertaken. You cannot thrive on dead food!

3. Ameliorate Digestion and Absorption

For many people this process is absolutely vital. Not only will improving digestion and absorption help with weight loss but it will dramatically improve your health as your body begins to actually absorb ALL and not just SOME nutrients.

As the saying goes…

"You are what you eat, but you are also what you digest and absorb!"

Wouldn't you agree that if you eat the healthiest, organic raw foods but cannot process and absorb them properly then you won't receive their full benefit?

The other pressing issue when it comes to improperly digested foods is the potential for the development of allergies. You can only ever be allergic to a protein (not a carbohydrate or fat), and this normally occurs as incompletely digested protein molecules seep out of the intestinal tract. Under optimal conditions, all food molecules are fully broken down and easily absorbed through their specific channels or "pores" in the intestinal tract. However, when larger, undigested protein molecules make their way through the intestines, they end up binding to the intestinal walls causing inflammation, irritation, and a subsequent widening of intestinal pores.

This condition is known as **Leaky Gut Syndrome**, and is characterized by increased permeability of the intestinal walls allowing undigested protein molecules into the blood stream. With these "unrecognizable" protein molecules traveling through the blood, your body then mounts an immune response against these food antigens that are seen as foreign invaders. Your body is simply doing what it knows how to do – fighting off unidentified floating objects. So you can see how important proper digestion is to the body!

Incomplete digestion throws the intestinal flora (bacteria) way out of balance as well. This alone could be the topic for an entire book.

Can you relate to any of these symptoms?

- Excessive gas, belching, or burping after meals?
- Stomach bloated after eating?
- Sleepy after eating?
- Longitudinal striations on fingernails?
- Eat when rushed/in a hurry?
- Bad breath?
- Full feeling after a heavy meat meal?
- Nausea after taking supplements?
- Acne?
- Undigested food in the stool?

If you answered YES to any of the symptoms, then you most likely have an underactive stomach (as does about 80% of the population) which means that, because your stomach has most likely been damaged from years of abuse, it no longer secretes adequate amounts of hydrochloric acid and digestive enzymes to fully break down your food. Your stomach has simply had enough! If you abuse it with terrible foods, it will no longer respond when you need it to. However, you can re-establish a trusting and loving relationship with your stomach and digestive system by feeding it whole living plant-based foods and following fundamental steps to reducing the stress you impose upon them.

As you can see, not digesting your foods properly can have profound effects on your body. By putting the following suggestions into action you will substantially improve your ability to digest and absorb your foods, and reduce the prevalence of the aforementioned symptoms.

1. **Chew Your Food –** very, very important!!!

   This is fairly obvious. Even our parents have always told us to chew our food before swallowing. I have friends whom I call "human vacuums" because they don't even chew their food at all. You turn your head for a minute and their food is gone! I'm sure you know people like that as well.

   There's an ancient Indian proverb that states: "Chew your food well, for the stomach has no teeth." How true is that!

   You should take your time when you eat. Chew your food thoroughly so that it mixes well with the digestive enzymes in your saliva. Before swallowing, the food in your mouth should feel like mush. Just another reason why animal meats are so hard on your body – they take forever to chew and most people don't even bother!

2. **Put Down Your Fork, Spoon, or Food Between Bites**

   This is another technique I find helpful in slowing me down when eating. By taking a bite, and putting your food or utensil down, you automatically allow your mouth to finish chewing before taking the next bite. Try it – it definitely slows things down but food is meant to be enjoyed. Don't rush it!

3. **Express Love and Gratitude Towards Your Food**

   Fully enjoying your food and being grateful for its presence is critical. When you eat, you don't just eat the food on your plate but you also take in all the energy around you at the time. By expressing gratitude for the food that you are eating, you put your body into a state of love and appreciation which greatly assists digestion. We've all experienced this. This even comes into play when preparing foods. By adding the magic ingredient "love" into the preparation, you transform the energy of the food making it highly absorbable in your body. Remember, everything is energy, and you are connected to everything because of this energy. You can shape everything around you, including food, through your thoughts and feelings.

I'm sure you've had an amazing meal at someone's house after which you tried to recreate on your own. If you're like me I'm sure you'll have noticed that it's never the same! Never! There's something missing – that special ingredient that for whatever reason cannot be explained.

Loving your food is also absolutely critical when eating LEISURE FOODS (or foods that are not great for you). Even if you eat an oily, fat-laden hamburger with all the toppings and French fries on the side, don't beat yourself up or feel guilty throughout the entire meal! Enjoy it! Yes, that's right, enjoy it! Your body will have a much easier time at processing the "garbage" you've just ingested. I've even heard some holistic nutritionists theorize that it could even be healthier to have a "non-healthy" meal and truly enjoy it, then eating a wonderfully "healthy" meal and hating every bite!

So eat well, be grateful for and enjoy your food. And do the exact same thing when you have your occasional splurge. Feelings of guilt, self-hatred, and any other negative feelings must be eliminated for they stress your body. When your body is stressed it doesn't digest.

4. Eat in a Soothing, Non-Stressful Environment

Eating while watching the news, eating with people who stress you out, eating on the run – these are all situations you want to avoid as best as possible. Why? When your body is stressed, blood is diverted away from the digestive tract and flows towards the muscles – meaning impoverished digestion. Remember the "Fight or Flight" response? The same process is at play here.

By eating in a soothing, relaxing environment you will dramatically help your body digest and assimilate the food you're eating. Put on some nice music, light a candle, and eat at the table instead of in front of the TV or computer.

5. Listen to Your Body – Stop When You're Full

This is self-evident yet many people have a problem with overeating and stuffing their faces until they turn blue. Practice moderation and don't eat past the point of satiety. By eating more whole living plant-based foods you'll actually find you won't need to eat as much because you'll be providing your body with all the nutrients it needs. Choose smaller plates or bowls. Use smaller glassware.

6. Practice Proper Food Combining

Food combining is the principle which holds that cooked proteins and cooked carbohydrates should not be eaten together. This is because carbohydrates require an alkaline environment (mouth, small intestine) for their digestion while proteins require an acidic environment (stomach, large intestine). Therefore, combining both in the same meal neutralizes their respective digestion environments and doesn't allow for optimal digestion.

Food combining has made an immense difference for me and I highly recommend it for most people. Although following a diet based on living plant foods will allow for more flexibility in food combining because of the inherent self-digesting capacity of raw foods, here are my **ABC's of Food Combining** (many of which come from David Wolfe's *Sunfood Diet Success System)* that I think will help...especially as you transition.

a. If cooked foods are eaten, try to eat only one type per meal and eat them with green vegetables.

b. Fruit is best eaten alone because it is highly enzymatic and self-digesting. You may try eating sweet fruits with green vegetables and/or healthy fats as long as no gas/flatulence is created. I personally enjoy mango and avocado together – but find what works best for your body.

c. If sweet fruits are eaten with cooked or steamed non-starchy vegetables (asparagus, broccoli, cauliflower), the fruit should be eaten first. In general, sweet fruits should not be mixed with cooked or dehydrated foods due to the potential for fermentation and gas.

d. It is best to eat one type of fruit at a time (mono-eating). As your digestive strength increases, you may wish to combine multiple types of fruit if your body allows.

e. Green leafy vegetables of different varieties may be eaten together.

f. Green leafy vegetables should always be eaten with any cooked starches (bread, pasta, rice, cakes).

g. Plant proteins (aka. Superfoods) such as hemp protein, goji berries, algae, and bee pollen may be eaten with light green vegetables such as lettuce and celery. They may also combine with sweet fruits and oils in smoothies as long as they do not produce any gas/flatulence.

h. Fiber-bound plant proteins such as spouted grains and legumes should be eaten with alkaline green vegetables to balance out their acids. Sprouted grains/legumes typically do not mix well with fats/oils and sweet fruits, although they seem to be ok for some people.

i. Animal proteins (except whey) do not mix well with fats/oils or sweet fruits and thus should be eaten with green leafy salads for additional fiber and alkalinity.

j. Low-sugar fruits (tomatoes, cucumbers) may be eaten together and combined with cruciferous vegetables (which can also be combined among different types).

k. Low-sugar fruits may be eaten with greens or fats, and can also be juiced with green vegetables.

l. Raw fermented foods (ie. sauerkraut) may be eaten with green leafy vegetables to calm their digestion as well as with cooked foods.

m. Raw cruciferous vegetables and sprouts are typically more bound up in fiber than other vegetables and may be difficult for some people to digest. Therefore, eating them with fruit may cause gas/flatulence due to the incomplete digestion of both foods. Instead, eat raw cruciferous vegetables and sprouts with green leafy vegetables and healthy fats.

n. Avoid drinking water and other liquids with your meals as it will dilute your stomach's acid and not allow full and proper digestion. If anything take little sips throughout your meal to add lubrication to drier foods. Drink lukewarm water 10-15 minutes before your meal and/or 15-20 minutes after your meal. Avoid drinking ice cold water before, during, or after food as the cold water will freeze shut your stomach's parietal glands, hindering the stomach's ability to digest.

o. For larger meals, begin with a lukewarm glass of lemon water (fresh squeezed lemon). This will stimulate stomach acid secretion and rev up your stomach for the upcoming food.

p. Avoid eating sweet foods (desserts, fruits) right after your meal because the sugar will quickly metabolize and ferment on top of the rest of the food that is still being processed. Gas/flatulence, bloating, and fatigue may result.

Do your best to follow these Food Combining ABC's. Doing so will greatly help your digestion, alleviate stress on your digestive system, and help your stomach build back its confidence and strength. As you transition further into eating raw living foods you will most likely experience the ability to bypass many of these guidelines as your digestive system will have greatly improved and because of the enzymes present in living whole foods. I personally found it rather easy to combine plant-based proteins, sweet fruits, and healthy fats/oils in a single meal after months of having adopted more of a raw foods diet.

4.   Reduce Your Stress

This may be one of the most important elements to a long and healthy life. Even though whole living foods can help you fend off stress to a certain degree, being able to manage and minimize your stress is vitally important. Because stress can be chemical/environmental, physical, emotional, and psychological it is important to look at strategies to decrease it in all areas.

<u>Reduce Chemical and Environmental Stress</u>

1. **Choose Locally Grown Organic Foods Whenever Possible**
    Foods that are non-organic are loaded with pesticide residues, fillers, preservatives, and who knows what else. Why would you put such chemicals in your body? Your body can only take so much toxic load before it wears down and exhibits disease. The liver is your body's main detoxifier and the more toxins it has to deal with the more compromised it will become. Furthermore, the more foreign agents you introduce into your body, the more the immune system is called into action. If your immune system is constantly bombarded and mounting immune responses to such chemicals, the quicker it will become fatigued, not function properly, and breakdown. This is when chronic diseases begin to surface.

    Unfortunately, organic foods are slightly more expensive, but if you can support local organic farmers, eventually those prices will come down. Do your best to choose organic especially with fruits and vegetables. If you don't have access to organic foods, be sure to thoroughly wash your fruits and vegetables (even with a light natural soap) to remove as much chemical residue as possible.

2. **Drink Only Purified Spring Water**
    Tap water, no matter how healthy authorities may claim it to be, is terrible. It is full of carcinogens like chlorine and fluoride, and trace amounts of antibiotic and medication residues from people flushing their medicines down the toilet! I

wouldn't even recommend distilled water as it is "dead water" and can actually leach valuable minerals from your body. Your best option is spring water as it contains all the elements nature intended for water and your body.

If you don't have access to spring water, then do your best to get either a reverse osmosis or carbon filtration system for your home.

When you're not at home and need to rely on bottled water, here are few things to look for:

  i. Glass bottle is best
  ii. The darker the bottle the better
  iii. If plastic, then make sure it is solid (not pliable) and darker in colour.

Remember that water is your lifeblood. You are almost entirely water, so choosing healthy living water can have a tremendous benefit to your health. In fact, the body can actually go for more than 30 days on nothing but water and still feel fully energized.

Reduce Physical Stress

1. **Inactivity is Stressful on the Body But So is Too Much Exercise!**
   I'll discuss this in more detail in the next chapter but for now realize that a healthy balance of moderate intensity exercise is necessary for a healthy, energized, and fit body. Never exercising or exercising too hard and too often can be very taxing on your adrenal glands - eventually wearing them down - and your immune system.

Reduce Emotional and Psychological Stress

This is the biggest and most powerful of all stressors. Stress is something that we impose upon ourselves most of the time. It is the projection of the "possibility" of a negative event in the future. It can also be caused by a feeling of overwhelm. You create your life. Your thoughts determine your feelings which in turn determine your actions. And since your actions yield specific results, it is important to go back to the source of the problem – your thoughts!

1. **Turn Down the "Mind-Frick"**

   What if I told you that you had 3 minutes to prepare a speech that you would give in front of 1,000 people immediately? For most people this would be a huge shock to the system and an immediate stressor. As you read this did you notice your mind saying certain things like "There's no way!", "I can't do that", and "I can't talk in front of large audiences!" These are non-empowering thoughts otherwise known as "mind-frick". It is important to recognize that these thoughts arise out of your conditioned mind – not your true self – which is based in fear and protection.

   Being aware of these negative thoughts is the first step in being able to change them. Realize that whether you think you can or can't do something, you're right. Your perception is your reality. It doesn't matter what anyone else thinks because if you firmly believe that you can't do something you won't.

   I have seen this so many times with clients. First of all I'm astonished at how little credit people give themselves and how little self-esteem most people have. For instance, I've asked clients of mine to perform push-ups on a stability ball only to hear "Oh, no...there's no way! I can never do that. Are you crazy?!" I reply by saying "YES! Yes I am crazy! But so are you for not believing in your own abilities!" The amazing part is that within 1 or 2 attempts they have almost perfected the movement!

As a fitness/nutrition/wellness coach my objective ultimately boils down to motivating and empowering you to take action with the tools that I provide to you. Most people know the importance of eating well and exercising yet so few actually walk the walk. The limiting factor in 98% of cases is the limiting and negative psychology that is poisoning peoples' minds.

So, I encourage you right now to make a list of limiting beliefs that you have about achieving whatever goals are important to you. Once you've established this list, I'd like you to take each statement or limiting belief and rephrase it in the positive, crossing out the negative one for good.

For instance, a limiting belief might be the following:
"I don't have time to exercise and prepare healthy foods"

This should be replaced with a positive statement like:
"I always create time to exercise and prepare healthy meals because I know that they are very important in helping me achieve my goals!"

By replacing negative self-talk with positive affirmations, your body and mind will automatically change toward the latter more often. Remember, everything in your external world started in your internal world. It started as a thought, a feeling. And according to the **Law of Attraction**, what you focus on expands so program your mind to focus on positive empowering thoughts instead of limiting, self-destructive, negative thoughts. The great news is that the choice is yours. The bad news is the choice is yours. Either way you have the power and control to choose which conversations occur in your head. I'll let you choose!

2. **Take Time Each Day to Meditate, Breathe, and Visualize**
   This is a very powerful process. Take at least 10-15 minutes either in the morning or at night (or both) to close your eyes, breathe, meditate, and visualize your life the way you would like it to be. If you have trouble meditating on your own then find a meditation centre or audio CD that can help you get into the state.

Getting your mind off the stresses and pressures of day-to-day living through these practices can have very powerful soothing effects on your body. Many scientific studies have shown this to be the case. Recently, a study published in **Psychosomatic Medicine** demonstrated that meditation changes brain and immune function in positive ways and contributes to greater health outcomes.[34]

When you sleep you automatically breathe, but you do not automatically eat. We survive for weeks without food, days without water, but only a few minutes without breathing! Breathing brings oxygen into your body and energizes it!

Proper breathing is so important – a few of its benefits include:

i. **The prevention of overeating**
   Simply by practicing some deep breathing before you eat can help you reduce the tendency to overeat.

ii. **Lymph drainage**
   Lymph (our body's sewage system) is 4x greater in volume than our blood and is crucial in keeping our immune system strong and healthy. As long as the lymph can circulate throughout the body via deep breathing and the action of the lungs, diaphragm, and intercostal muscles, it can be kept clean and help keep your body energized and strong.

iii. **Deep breathing alkalizes your body by removing carbonic acid.**

iv. **Longevity**

---

[34] Davidson, R. et al. (2003). Alterations in brain and immune function produced by mindulness meditation. *Psychosomatic Medicine*, 65: 564-570.

Species that breathe deeply and slowly tend to live the longest. Remember that energy expenditure and longevity are inversely related. The giant tortoise breathes only 4 times per minute, while humans breathe about 18 times per minute. The giant tortoise is one of the longest living animals on the planet.

Deep Breathing Technique

When you're ready to unwind, meditate, or simply de-stress you will find deep breathing to be of great benefit. Try using the following breathing ratio: 1:4:2. The means that you inhale for 1, hold for 4, and release for 2. I suggest you multiply this ratio by at least 3 times so that you actually inhale for 3 seconds, hold the breath for 12 seconds, and slowly release for 6 seconds. The longer you can extend the ratios, the more benefit you will receive from this exercise. Repeat for several minutes until you feel your state become more relaxed, centered, and liberated. This is a very relaxing method of breathing that can literally be done anywhere!

Energizing Breathing Technique

At times when you need a boost of energy the following breathing pattern is extremely effective. I personally use this every morning when I walk. The key component to this breathing method is that you must be moving – not sedentary. It helps stimulates blood flow, oxygen delivery, mental focus, and clarity!

With this energy breathing pattern what you're going to do is take 4 inhalations through your nose while tapping your thumb to each one of your fingers (ie. of the same hand - thumb to index, thumb to middle finger, etc... ending on the pinky) so each breath in corresponds to a particular thumb/finger tap.

Once you've reached the 4th inhalation (thumb-pinky tap), you will then begin your exhalation in a mirroring 4 breath "out" pattern, again applying the thumb-finger tap method. Be sure to exhale through your mouth. Repeat this sequence for several minutes and you'll feel your state transform!

As you perform your breathing, relaxation, or meditation exercises you can use empowering visualization to further bring great results into your life. Visualize what you want to create. See yourself as you'd like to look and feel. Put a smile on your face. It is impossible to feel sad, depressed or stressed when you think positive thoughts and maintain a smile on your face!

5. Exercise on a Regular Basis

We all know that regular exercise is essential to a long and healthy life. It reduces the risk of pretty much all disease, strengthening your body's immune system, cardiovascular system, and musculoskeletal structure. It helps improve your posture, increases the quality of your sleep and prevents fat gain which leaves you feeling energized and more confident.

Considering these benefits, why is it that so many people cannot make exercise part of their lifestyle? I'll tell you why. Most people associate too much pain to the process of exercising and maintain focus on the possibility of pain. This consumes their thoughts entirely. They never focus on the amazing outcomes they know they are going to experience shortly thereafter. Having worked with thousands of individuals from all walks of life, I can attest that those who succeed and make exercise a habit are those that focus on the goals that they want to achieve. Let's be honest, exercise can be a terrible process for many people. You've got to sweat, push your body out of its comfort zone, and do things that you would not normally consider doing. But that's also why it's such an empowering tool. Exercise can instill confidence and a sense of accomplishment like nothing else. The key is to focus on the end result!

I've received some of the most amazing testimonials from my clients around the world whose lives have been changed by my one-on-one coaching or my audio guided workout programs, like Fitter U™. It is an absolutely phenomenal feeling to positively impact peoples' lives. If you don't exercise regularly, then start! If you exercise on a regular basis or are a high level athlete, then keep it up!

If you are brand new to exercise and don't know where to start then you can follow the 4 step process I have outlined for you below. If you still need more structure, motivation, and guidance, then I highly recommend you get started with my 12-week Fitter U™ program. Visit **www.myFitterU.com** to learn more about how Fitter U™ can help you.

In the meantime, you can start getting active by following these steps:

Step #1 - Walk at Least 30 Minutes Every Day!

Walking is one the most beneficial activities you can adopt. It is low stress on the body and has tremendous benefits when it comes to building an aerobic foundation, reducing body fat, and maintaining adequate range of motion in your joints.

Walk whenever you have the chance be it to work, to the store, or anywhere else. Grab a partner or join a walking group to give you some extra motivation and accountability.

Step #2 - Engage in Moderate Intensity Aerobic Training 2-4x per Week

Walking is a great start but you also have to ensure that you're pushing your cardiovascular system a little more than normal. Instead of using your heart rate as a gauge (many people find this tedious) you can use what I call the **"Talk Test"**. The Talk Test ensures that you can carry a conversation while exercising. This would be appropriate for your walking.

But now that you want to step up the intensity, you need to get to a point where **maintaining a conversation is no longer easy to do**. You're beginning to hear that "huff and puff" of your breathing. Choose any cardio/aerobic activity that you enjoy - running, biking, elliptical, swimming, sports, etc...

You want to do this type of cardio/aerobic training 2-4 times per week for at least 20 minutes. Visit **www.myTreadmillTrainer.com** and **www.EllipticalWorkouts.com** to get the best cardio workouts available!

Step #3 - Strength Train 2-4x per Week

Resistance (or strength) training is absolutely critical to developing lean muscle and burning fat. It will dramatically increase your resting metabolic rate, strengthen and support your joints, and leave you feeling strong and energetic.

This type of training can take the form of body weight exercises (ie. push-ups, pull-ups, lunges, crunches, dips, etc...) or any other method which will stress your muscles (ie. free weights, tubing, etc...).

These workouts should be well balanced and attend to the body's full musculature. They do not necessarily have to be broken up into "chest-biceps" types of routines either. I prefer using full-body functional training which means training movements, not muscle groups. This is the most effective way to develop total body strength, balance between muscle groups, and to assist in weight loss.

For starters, choose 6 exercises and do 3 sets of each for 10-15 reps with a weight that will challenge you by the last few reps.

Step #4 - Stretch on a Daily Basis (and especially after exercise)

Stretching is crucial in order to maintain muscle flexibility and fluid body motion. The last thing you want is to be strong and have great musculature but limited in your range of motion (especially for athletes). Having a good degree of flexibility is also correlated with a reduction in injuries.

Stretching after (not before) your exercise sessions is recommended and helpful in restoring normal muscle length, especially since the muscles have just been subjected to increased loads and have most likely built up a good amount of toxins (ie. lactic acid).

Hold your stretches for 20-30 seconds (without bouncing) and breathe deeply to help further the stretch and deliver oxygen to the muscles. Activities like yoga are great for keeping the body limber.

Once again, if all this seems a little overwhelming or if you're looking for greater results from your workouts, then my Fitter U™ program will definitely help. **Visit www.myFitterU.com for more information on getting started.**

Nutrition
for ATHLETES

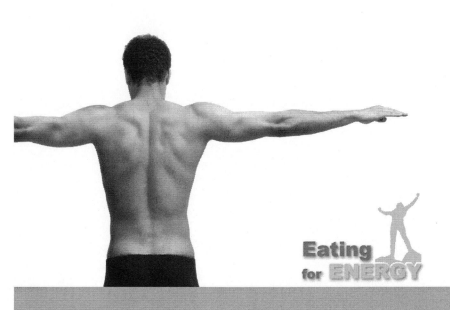

Eating
for ENERGY

Nutrition for Athletes

The value of natural, high-quality nourishment is appreciated by the nutritionally savvy athlete. Without proper nutrition it is very difficult to achieve your full physical potential in your sport. However, the amazing thing is that about 80% of athletes somehow manage to get by in their respective sports with poor nutritional habits. It blows my mind! Just imagine how much better their performance could be if they improved their eating habits.

I used to train a handful of high level hockey players, from the NCAA (college) level right up to the NHL (professional). One of the "pros" who truly stood out above the rest was in his mid 30's and made it his mission to fully understand how nutrition and conditioning could transform his body and thus his performance. I remember asking him if his "colleagues" had the same level of knowledge and application when it came to eating well and he replied "Absolutely not!" He went on to tell me that many pro hockey players had no clue and that their eating habits were atrocious.

My own experience in soccer confirms these reports. I remember having teammates who would be drinking coffee one hour before a game on a blistering hot day! Not only that, we even had some players who smoked! It is truly amazing how the body somehow finds a way to perform under such conditions.

All elite athletes eventually come to appreciate that the most crucial element for building athletic performance lies in their ability to recover. Without a doubt this is the most important aspect of performance. Being able to train every day of the week, sometimes twice a day, and still manage to improve your performance without injuries is not an easy task. Now perhaps you don't train as hard or as often as most pro athletes but the fact still remains that your body is always under some level of stress be it physical, emotional, or environmental. All of these stressors will eventually wear down your body, and hence your ability to perform to the best of your ability. As we have discussed in this book, living plant-based foods have far greater nutrient density, greater amounts of enzymes, and are much more easily processed by your body. They should make up at least 80% of your diet. As a once meat-eating professional athlete to an almost completely raw vegan avid exerciser and health promoter, I have noticed a night and day difference in all areas of my health and performance as I have gotten away from commonly held "mis-beliefs" of what does a body good, and adopted a way of eating that actually works!

In general, the closer your workouts are to each other, the quicker you will improve but only if you provide your body with the nourishment it requires. Your ability to recover quickly and bounce back for the next training session or competition will depend on how you fuel your body and the degree to which it can rest and repair. If it can do so, the performance gains will be unmistakable. Whether you're a high level or a recreational athlete the same rules apply. Quick cellular repair is paramount. If you eat health promoting foods after exercise, your body will not have to dedicate as much energy to recovery as it might otherwise need to if you ate poorly. Proper nutrition allows your body's other important systems such as the immune and hormonal systems to remain in better health. For instance, one of the signs of overtraining is an increased susceptibility to infection and sickness. This occurs because so much energy is being spent on regenerating your body that the immune system becomes so overworked that it can no longer perform its functions of fending off disease and keeping microorganisms at bay.

It is important to understand which nutrients will allow you to perform and recover most effectively, as well as when you should eat relative to your workouts. Remember that the body needs a combination of carbohydrates, amino acids (protein), healthy fats, water, and an array of vitamins and minerals to do its job. The following section will detail what to eat and drink before, during, and after your exercise session.

The timing of nutrition combined with specifically formulated recipes for athletic performance is crucial. The following will go into detail about how applying a living plant-based diet will help you perform greater than ever before!

Eating before Exercise

The first thing to understand, from a fuel perspective, is that your body will tap into meals you consumed a day prior much more effectively than a pre-exercise meal or snack. The reason for this is that it takes time for the body to digest, absorb, and then restore necessary energy reserves.

So if you go for a run on Saturday morning, the main fuel source for that run will be derived from what you ate the night and day prior, not necessarily what you had for breakfast.

This is an important concept to remember since many people think they can get away with polluting their body for several days and then all of a sudden eat a healthy pre-exercise meal and everything will be ok. That just doesn't happen.

Your body is an accumulation of nutrients that you have consumed over the years. Are you built of pizza or energizing living plant-based foods? The difference is night and day. All that being said, it is helpful to have a nutritious pre-exercise snack or meal to top up your energy reserves before getting started.

Your body's first choice of fuel during exercise is carbohydrates. Carbohydrates are stored in the body as glycogen, both in the liver and muscle. The liver's job is to break down glycogen into glucose to maintain suitable levels of glucose in the blood. The muscles on the other hand, tap directly into their glycogen stores for energy production.

Depending on the duration and intensity of the exercise, your body will rely on more complex carbohydrates (stored as glycogen in the muscles and liver) and fatty acids for its fuel.

The following graph shows the relationship between **exercise intensity and energy used from different fuel sources**.

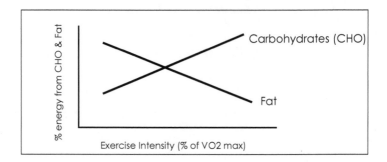

Notice that as the intensity of exercise increases, there is more reliance on carbohydrates for fuel. Typically, intensities greater than 70% of VO2 max (or maximum heart rate for our purposes) will have carbohydrates as the dominant fuel source. However, this doesn't mean that working at high intensities doesn't burn fat. Working at higher intensities allows more total calories to be burned and that's what really matters if you're looking to lose weight.

Compare the intensity graph with this next graph showing the relationship between **exercise duration and fuel selection**:

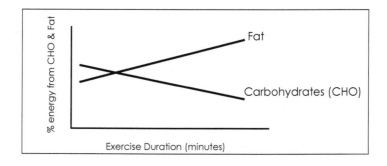

It's pretty much the opposite isn't it?

The point is that your body chooses different fuels during different situations. Because fats yield more calories and are slower burning as they are metabolized, they tend to be used over longer durations when compared to carbohydrates. However, the body wants to conserve its blood glucose and glycogen stores. As you become fitter your body will become more efficient at using fats for fuel while sparing your vital carbohydrate reserves. Someone who is totally unfit will obviously fatigue sooner, one of the reasons being that their carbohydrate stores are more quickly dissolved and utilized. Fitter individuals can last much longer because they have developed the ability to use the slow burning fats as fuel, and therefore conserve their energy better.

Carbohydrates that are used during exercise come from both glycogen stores in muscle and from blood glucose. Within carbohydrate metabolism blood glucose and glycogen are used to varying degrees depending on the nature of the activity. However, the body's first order of business is in maintaining healthy blood glucose levels. Blood glucose is the main fuel source for the brain, so I'm sure you can appreciate why it's pretty important. As intensity increases, muscle glycogen is increasingly used. Blood glucose use also increases slightly. However, to offset its usage and to maintain stable blood sugar levels (for the vital organs), the liver breaks down its glycogen stores into glucose for the blood.

So, after giving you a rather lengthy lesson in exercise physiology and bioenergetics, all that you have to remember is the bulk of your pre-exercise meal/snack should come from complex carbohydrates (CHO). Eating too much protein before exercise will likely lead to cramping since protein requires more water to be metabolized than does CHO or fat.

Also protein is not a very good fuel source – it's meant for building your body, not fueling it. Also, when protein is used as fuel instead of CHO, it burns "dirty", meaning that toxins are created from its combustion. The production and elimination of toxins are a stress on the body and cause a stress response leading to a decline in endurance.

Here are some general **pre-exercise guidelines** that should help you:

1. Pre-exercise feeding should contain 1 to 5 grams of CHO/kg of body weight, and should be taken 3 to 4 hours before exercise.

2. The CHO source should be an easily digestible solid complex CHO food, but if taken 1 hour before exercise, it should be in liquid or gel form.

3. As an athlete, you should test these feeding protocols in training before using them in competition.

I mentioned earlier that topping up your glycogen stores with a pre-exercise snack is a good idea. But as you can imagine there is a difference between someone who works out in the gym and someone who runs a marathon. So there must be varying energizing "snack" protocols to address these needs. I've separated these protocols into 2 separate categories.

Type I Activities: High intensity, shorter duration (lasting less than 1 hour)

Examples: 3 to 6 mile run, intense gym workout, tennis, sprinting, basketball

Type II Activities: moderate intensity, longer duration (lasting 1 to 3 hours)

Examples: half marathon, marathon, longer cycling events, hiking, soccer/hockey/tennis matches that last more than 1 hour.

Type I Activities – Pre-Exercise Snack Ideas

For short bouts of high-intensity exercise, fuel up on simple carbohydrates. The healthiest source of these is fruit. **Dates** are your best choice since they are rich in glucose, the basic sugar molecule that goes straight to the liver for immediate energy, meaning your body doesn't waste precious energy converting it from another form in order to utilize it. However, glucose burns quickly which means that if glucose is your only carbohydrate source, it will need to be replenished every 20 minutes if your exercise session lasts more than 1 hour, to keep you going strong. The influx of glucose into the blood means that your blood glucose levels will be maintained for longer periods of time, thus reducing the onset of fatigue while maximizing your performance.

Another great source of energy comes from fructose – fruit sugar. All fruits (bananas, mangos, oranges, etc...) contain fructose. Fructose is less quick to metabolize because it first needs to be converted to glucose by the liver. As a result, it has a lower glycemic index than glucose, meaning that it kicks in at a slower rate once ingested, and burns more slowly. One of the great sources of fructose is **agave nectar** (from the blue agave cactus, the same source of tequila), a wonderful natural sweetener. It adds sweetness to foods yet does not have a strong taste or a lingering after-taste (ie. unlike stevia).

Now, I'm really going to cause some turmoil! One of the best sources of fuel for exercise is coconut oil! Yes that's right, coconut oil. Coconut oil is a tremendous source of medium-chain triglycerides (MCTs) which are chemically much different from both short and long-chain triglycerides found in other foods. MCTs are actually more similar to carbohydrates than fats in regards to how they are processed by the body. Most fats get stored as fat if not used for energy right away. However, MCTs are highly thermogenic (raise the body temperature and cellular activity) and go directly to the liver where they are metabolized and used as instant energy! Furthermore, the water that is found inside the coconut is nature's natural sports drink. Coconut water contains an almost identical electrolyte composition to your body's interstitial fluid, serving as a healthy and natural hydrator which will undoubtedly enhance your performance.

Type II Activities – Pre-Exercise Snack Ideas

If you're going to be exercising for several hours, you'll want to consume a few more sustainable sources of energy in addition to the glucose, fructose, and MCT recommendations from Type I activities. You'll also want to add a small amount of alkaline protein such as hemp or whey and some essential fatty acids like fish/flax seed oil or even some ground flaxseeds or ground soaked almonds for more prolonged and sustained energy.

Fuel during Exercise

As we've already mentioned, glucose is very quickly depleted during moderate to intense activity. Therefore, if you are exercising for more than 1 hour, your performance can be enhanced and fatigue delayed by ingesting some quickly absorbable glucose-based fuels. It is best to get these fuels in liquid form (ie. sport drinks) or in gels and puddings. This is not the time to be eating solid foods. You want your body to direct its energy towards physical performance, not digestion.

Sport Drinks are definitely the best option in long duration conditions. And I'm not talking about your standard corn syrup-based, dye-infused garbage! I have listed several natural sport drink recipes in the *"Hydration and Exercise"* section just a few pages on to give you some healthy hydration alternatives.

Puddings and sport gels are just that – mushy like concoctions that contain quickly absorbable sugars and performance sustaining nutrients such as essential fatty acids, MCTs, and even small amounts of amino acids. As a base most of them contain glucose-rich dates and easily digestible fruits like bananas. Agave nectar is also included for its fructose content. Here are a couple of recipes that you can sneak in during half-time, while running, or at a pit stop. These gels/puddings can be stored in a plastic bag or gel flasks (which can be bought at most athletic/running stores). Whether the snack becomes a gel or pudding really depends on how much liquid you add to it – do whatever is best for you!

These gels and puddings also make great pre-exercise snacks. If you need something quick and energizing before your exercise session, then grab one of these recipes 1 hour before you start and you'll be good to go.

Sport Gels and Puddings

Preparation: Add all ingredients into a blender or food processor and process until smooth.

Mint Chocolate Gel

4 dates, pre-soaked

2 tbsp agave nectar

2 tsp of raw cacao powder

Juice of ½ lemon

1 tsp lemon zest

Pinch of sea salt

1 tsp dried mint

High Octane

5 dates, pre-soaked

2 tbsp coconut oil

½ banana

2 tsp lemon zest

1 tsp lemon juice

Pinch of sea salt

Chocolate Monkey

1 banana

5 dates, pre-soaked

2 tbsp ground flaxseed

1 tbsp ground sesame seed

2 tsp raw cacao powder

1 tbsp coconut oil

1 tsp lemon juice

Pinch of sea salt

Blue-Green Gel

1 banana

4 dates, pre-soaked

1 tbsp spirulina

¼ cup blueberries

1 tbsp ground flaxseed

1 tbsp coconut oil

Pinch of sea salt

Post Workout Pudding

2 bananas

1 cup blueberries

½ cup soaked almonds

2 tbsp ground flaxseeds

1 tbsp ground sesame seeds

2 tbsp hemp or whey protein powder

1 tbsp raw cacao powder

1 tsp lemon juice

Pinch of sea salt

1 tbsp fish or flax seed oil

Post-Exercise Nutrition

Post workout nutrition is vital to your healthy body. In order to recover properly your body needs essential nutrients to rebuild and re-energize. You've worked hard in the gym, completed your run, or just finished an intense game and don't want your sweat and effort to go unrewarded, right? Well, the following information is essential in assuring you get the most from your training and able your body to recover the best it can.

It is important to realize that making poor food choices following exercise will reduce the benefits of exercise, weaken your immune system, increase the likelihood of injury, cause hypoglycemia (drop in blood sugar) and reduce your energy and performance during subsequent exercise sessions.

Carbohydrates, proteins and healthy fats all have an important role in the post exercise nutrition. While working out or exercising, your body mainly uses muscle glycogen and blood glucose as its main fuel sources. These glycogen and blood sugar levels can be severely depleted upon completion of an intense workout and must be replenished shortly thereafter to ensure proper recovery.

Exercise, and specifically weight lifting, causes microtears in the muscle fibers (protein degradation). This is what causes muscle soreness but also what stimulates their recovery to a stronger state than before. Since muscles are made up of protein, post-workout protein consumption is important to foster quick and full regeneration.

I also highly recommend adding essential fatty acids for the role they play in reducing inflammation, supporting the immune system, and building healthy cell membranes.

Another component I recommend adding to a post-exercise smoothie is Maca. Maca is an ancient Peruvian root vegetable that has tremendous adrenal supporting benefits. Considering that intense exercise places significant stress on the adrenal glands, maca can play a noteworthy role in helping your body come back to balance and reduce its stress load. Maca powder is the easiest form to use.

After your exercise session, fuel replenishment (glycogen stores), muscle regeneration, and rehydration (discussed later) are your three main goals. As such, food choices that stimulate the release of insulin (ie. sugars) will cause the most effective uptake of carbohydrates into the muscles. This increase in insulin levels due to consuming carbohydrates after exercise also increases muscle repair because insulin stimulates muscle protein synthesis. High quality protein and essential fatty acids will foster proper recovery of muscle tissue and other cellular damage, respectively. The quicker you can get the proper nutrients into your body after your workout, the more effective your recovery will be. By ensuring those nutrients come from plant-based whole foods, you will greatly assist your recovery.

The ideal is to consume a quickly absorbable (high glycemic index) form of carbohydrates within 15 minutes of your workout's end. This can take the form of a sport drink, fruit juice, fruit, or the sport gels and puddings. After this initial glucose-rich drink/snack, you can have a more substantial smoothie that balances carbohydrate-rich foods with high quality alkalizing proteins (hemp or whey) and essential fatty acids. Whey protein has been found to stimulate the release of insulin. Therefore, it would be an effective protein to consume after an exercise bout as the extra boost of insulin will help drive nutrients into the muscle cells. Whey protein is also a very high-quality protein that would help muscles recover more quickly. You can throw in some Maca if you like as well.

After your smoothie, it is preferable to have a more balanced and substantial meal no later than 2 hours post workout. As with your smoothie, this meal should contain good sources of carbohydrates, proteins, and essential fatty acids. Remember that you want to choose whole living plant-based foods for they have tremendous life force, contain huge amounts of enzymes, and are mostly alkaline forming in the body.

Hydration and Exercise

Hydration and performance go hand in hand. If your body is dehydrated it will fatigue faster and you suffer greatly. Staying well hydrated is especially important when exercising in hot environments. Total body water can have a critical influence on thermoregulation (the body's ability to maintain an acceptable temperature) and exercise performance, especially in the heat. Hypohydration (total body water below normal) has been attributed to high sweat rates, and therefore fluid loss, compounded by inadequate rehydration, or simply an initial pre-exercise water deficit.

Sweat rates, in athletes performing vigorous exercise in the heat, have been known to reach 1 – 2 L/h. During soccer matches, one investigator found sweat rates to reach 1.5 liters per game under cool conditions (10-15°C) and 3.5 to 4 liters per game under hot conditions (30-38°C).[35]

With increasing sweat loss athletic performance is significantly disturbed. Studies have shown performance and cognitive impairments to occur with fluid deficits as low as 1.8% and 2% of body mass.

In order to prevent hypohydration during exercise (especially in the heat), proper hydration strategies need to be implemented. Although much research has been done in this field, many coaches, athletes, and recreational exercisers are ignorant of the importance of proper hydration before, during, and after exercise. According to leading investigators in this field, daily fluid requirements (for sedentary to very active people) can range from 8 – 16 L/day![36] The researchers also identified the need to replace each liter of fluid lost with a subsequent liter of ingested fluid to maintain a normal hydration status. Therefore, 1 liter of sweat needs to be replaced by at least 1 liter of fluids.

---

[35] Shepherd, R. (1999). Minimizing the practical problems of world-wide soccer competition: management of heat exposure and a shift in circadian rhythms. Sci Sports. 14: 248-253.

[36] Latzka, W. and Montain, S. (1999). Water and electrolyte requirements for exercise. Clin. Sports. Med. 18: 513 – 524.

Having said that, taking in fluid during exercise may not fully prevent a fluid deficit. Most athletes typically only replace between 30-70% of the sweat losses they incurred during exercise. Therefore, as an athlete or recreational exerciser you should take several extra gulps beyond what satisfies your thirst. Remember that when it comes to thirst "If you're thirsty it's already too late!"

The following are recommendations made by the **American College of Sports Medicine** to help prevent the onset of dehydration and to optimize performance in hot environments.[37]

- **At least 2 hours prior to exercise, you should consume 500 ml of fluid**. This promotes proper hydration and allows time for the kidneys to excrete excess water, if any exists.
- **During exercise, you should begin consuming fluids at a rate equal to your sweat rate**. In general, this amounts to 150-200 ml every 15-20 min for most individuals.
- **Fluids should be cool (15-22°C), palatable, and readily available.**

Sodium is an essential electrolyte that is lost when you sweat. Sodium losses in sweat vary markedly between individuals but overall range from 20 – 80 mmol/L and depend on genetics, diet, sweat rate, hydration level, and heat acclimation state. Since an excessive sweat response in hot environments causes a significant loss of sodium and other electrolytes (ie. potassium, chloride), it is imperative to replenish these electrolytes during and after exercise (especially for durations longer than 1 hour). Commercial sport drinks are okay but from a natural nutrition perspective they're not the best solution because they contain artificial colouring, corn syrup, and other unnecessary additives.

Natural electrolyte solutions such as coconut water are wonderful healthy alternatives. Throw in a bit of agave nectar and a squeeze of lemon and lime juice for added alkalinity and you've just created a natural and delicious sports drink! Refer to the recipes below for full details on these natural sports drinks. Having one of these natural hydrators (or another sports drink if you don't have access to such ingredients) can be helpful in

---

[37] American College of Sports Medicine (1996). Position stand. Exercise and fluid replacement. *Medicine and Science in Sports and Exercise*, 28(1): i-vii.

preventing the deleterious effects of electrolyte imbalance (ie. hyponatremia – low sodium levels) and dehydration by providing optimal electrolyte and carbohydrate concentrations.

Sports drinks are beneficial in situations where exercise is performed for long durations (> 1 hour), and when exercising in hot environments. I wouldn't recommend them for anything less than an hour. I recommend that my clients get some simple sugars back into their body after a heavy workout, in the form of fruits, fruit juices, or natural sport drinks (described below).

If you are engaged in long-duration sporting activities, then sports drinks should have an optimal amount of carbohydrates (5-6% = 14g per 8oz) to give the working muscles more energy to help fight fatigue and provide better cognitive function. Research has shown that more than a 6% carbohydrate solution is not better since higher carbohydrate concentrations take longer to absorb and won't further enhance performance. Most likely, sports drinks with greater than a 6% carbohydrate concentration will lead to nothing more than stomach cramps.

Instead of commercial sports drinks try these natural alternatives for optimal hydration and performance.

Below the following recipe section you will find a 1-page "Hydration Protocol" chart that details for you the timing, quantities, and types of fluid to consume when exercising.

Natural Sport Drinks

Preparation: Add all ingredients into a blender and process until smooth. For Basic Sport Drink simply stir all ingredients in a glass.

Tropical Body Replenisher

1 cup coconut water

1 cup water

2 tbsp agave nectar

Juice of ½ lemon

Juice of ½ lime

Basic Sport Drink

3 cups fresh squeezed fruit juice

1 cup water

Pinch of sea salt

Citrus-Coconut Sport Drink

Juice of ½ lemon

Juice of ½ lime

2 dates, pre-soaked

2 cups water

1 cup coconut water

1 tbsp agave nectar

1 tsp coconut oil

Pinch of sea salt

Mint Chocolate Breeze

2 dates

2 cups water (or coconut water)

1 tbsp agave nectar

2 tsp of raw cacao powder

1 tsp dried mint

1 tsp coconut oil

Pinch of sea salt

Hydration Protocols

Exercise Duration	Timing of Consumption	Amount and Type
< 1 hr	**Before Exercise:** 1 – 2 hrs 15 – 30 min **During Exercise:** Every 10 – 15 min **Recovery:**	16 oz – cold water (CW) 10 – 16 oz CW or Sport Drink 6 – 8 oz CW adequate fluid to replace body weight losses
From 1 – 4 hrs	**Before Exercise:** 1 – 2 hrs 15 – 30 min **During Exercise:** Every 10 – 15 min **Recovery:**	16 oz Sport Drink or Water 10 – 16 oz Sport Drink 6 – 8 oz Sport Dink Immediately after and every 2 hrs Sport Drink to provide 1 g CHO/kg of body weight. Gel CHO and protein may also be used.
> 4 hrs	**Before Exercise:** 1 – 2 hrs 15 – 30 min **During Exercise:** Every 10 – 15 min **Recovery:** Immediately after and every 2 hrs	10 – 16 oz Sport Drink (5-10% CHO) 10 – 16 oz Sport Drink 6 – 8 oz Sport Drink + ½ tsp Sea Salt Immediately after and every 2 hrs Sport Drink to provide 1 g CHO/kg of body weight. Gel CHO and protein may also be used.

12-Week
meal PLAN

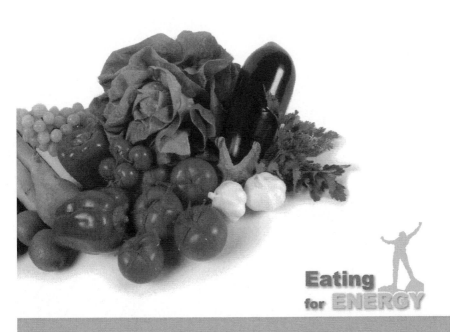

Eating
for ENERGY

The *Eating for Energy* 12-Week Meal Plan

The goal of this 12-week meal plan is to include significantly more raw plant foods into your diet. However, it is important to slowly transition into it since eating all raw may not be easy. Even though all the meals listed below are raw living foods, feel free to incorporate other dishes as you see fit. But do your best to keep it 80% raw! What follows is a Monday to Friday meal-by-meal dietary plan. On the weekends, feel free to eat other foods or pick some of your favourite recipes from the Healthy Recipe Guide. Although it is specific and structured, it is only a guide. If you don't feel like following it 100% or can't for whatever reason then that's fine. Do what works for you. It is meant to provide you with step-by-step guidance if that's what you're looking for; however, feel free to take some of these recipes and create your own meal schedule or even follow a few days of the meal plan and then eat other foods. I would rather you feel empowered and knowledgeable to make healthy decisions on your own.

Depending on your goals, you may also wish to incorporate more or fewer foods than what's described in the meal plan. Listen to your body. If you feel hungry and need more nutrients and calories, then add them. If you feel like there's too much food, then simply eat what you feel like eating and omit the rest.

By following this 12-week meal plan you will begin to notice astounding changes. You will notice more energy, improved body composition, glowing skin, greater mental clarity, improved athletic performance, and much more!

The goal is to see this way of eating as providing abundance rather than denial of the foods you enjoy. Feel free to include some of your favourite leisure foods as you begin to transition, but over time, the idea is to retrain your taste buds to no longer crave nutrient void foods. Be sure to give yourself 3-4 days between eating the same foods.

One of the central themes of this meal plan is variety and rotation. This concept is part of your Success Habits and is critically important. Variety will provide a wide range of nutrients to your body and prevent the development of addictions and food allergies. When you have the choice of smoothies, juices, or simply fruit, be sure not to drink/eat the same one at each occasion. Your body can become sensitive to any food if it is consistently exposed to it. So remember to choose from the wide array of recipes and foods that are at your disposal.

Most importantly, no matter what you eat be sure to fully enjoy it! Be grateful for your food and love every bite.

Don't forget to start your day with a glass of lukewarm water with the juice of ½ lemon (freshly squeezed).

To obtain the recipes for all the meals described in the Meal Plan simply turn to the Healthy Recipe Guide and Smoothie and Juice Guide.

May you enjoy these meals and begin to flourish with abundant energy and glowing health!

Week 1

Monday

Breakfast	Smoothie (your choice)
Snack	1 Apple with ¼ handful almonds and pumpkin seeds
Lunch	Waldorf salad
Snack	Guacamole with cucumber and bell peppers
Dinner	Creamy carrot ginger soup

Tuesday

Breakfast	Blue-Green Orange Bliss
Snack	Small handful goji berries and raw cacao nibs
Lunch	A date with Kale (6-10 wraps)
Snack	Hummus with broccoli, cauliflower, and celery
Dinner	Yammy's pad thai

Wednesday

Breakfast	Blueberry Morning
Snack	Selection of fresh berries
Lunch	Curry kale salad
Snack	Fresh pressed juice (your choice)
Dinner	Fettuccini cheddar pasta

Thursday

Breakfast   Fresh Pressed Green Juice (your choice)

Snack   Sunset Pudding

Lunch   Nori Wrap (side of Olive Tapenade optional)

Snack   Lentil Hummus with broccoli, cauliflower, and celery

Dinner   Zucchini Pasta with Marinara Sauce

Friday

Breakfast   Morning Muesli

Snack   Fruit with ¼ handful of almonds, walnuts, pumpkin seeds

Lunch   Popeye's Spinach and Herb Soup

Snack   Fresh pressed juice (your choice)

Dinner   Veggie Sushi with Spicy Mayonnaise

Week 2

Monday

Breakfast   Smoothie (your choice)

Snack   1 pear with ¼ handful almonds and sunflower seeds

Lunch   Broccoli soup

Snack   Chocolate Mousse

Dinner   Sweet Potato Pasta with Pesto Sauce

Tuesday

Breakfast   Porridge of Champions

Snack   Small handful goji berries and raw cacao nibs

Lunch   A date with Kale (6-10 wraps)

Snack   Lentil Hummus with broccoli, cauliflower, and celery

Dinner   Salad Slaw with Marinated Broccoli

Wednesday

Breakfast   Fresh Pressed Green Juice (your choice)

Snack   ¼ handful walnuts, pumpkin seeds, raisins

Lunch   Mango and Avocado Salad and Cream of Tomato Soup

Snack   Chocolate Energy Pudding

Dinner   Green Beans and Brown Rice in Curry Sauce

Thursday

Breakfast	Blueberry Morning
Snack	A Date with Kale
Lunch	Nori Wrap with Mango Chutney
Snack	Fresh Pressed Green Juice (your choice)
Dinner	Everything in the Fridge Salad

Friday

Breakfast	Morning Muesli
Snack	Smoothie (your choice)
Lunch	Corn and Lentil Salad
Snack	Strawberry – Banana Gelato
Dinner	Veggie Sushi with Spicy Mayonnaise

Week 3

Monday

Breakfast   Raw Oatmeal

Snack   Green veggies with Lentil Hummus

Lunch   Collard Taco with Tomato Salsa

Snack   Fresh Pressed Green Juice (your choice)

Dinner   Arugula Salad

Tuesday

Breakfast   Fresh Pressed Green Juice (your choice)

Snack   ½ handful of fresh coconut meat

Lunch   Waldorf Salad

Snack   Pistachio Halvah

Dinner   Salad from the Sea

Wednesday

Breakfast   Blueberry Morning

Snack   Spirulina (mixed with water or juice)

Lunch   Quinoa Paella

Snack   Raw chocolate (1 to 2 small bars)

Dinner   Green Beans and Brown Rice in Curry Sauce

Thursday

Breakfast   Smoothie (your choice)

Snack   Fresh Pressed Green Juice (your choice)

Lunch   Nori Wrap with Mango Chutney

Snack   Fresh Pressed Green Juice (your choice)

Dinner   Thai Salad

Friday

Breakfast   Morning Muesli

Snack   Smoothie (your choice)

Lunch   Carrot Salad

Snack   Lentil Hummus with Veggies

Dinner   Quinoa Salad with Mashed Potatoes

Week 4

The purpose of Week 4 is to gently cleanse your body. Although eating according this Meal Plan over the last 3 weeks has been greatly alkalizing and cleansing for your body, Week 4 introduces much more alkalinity and energy through green juices and salads. You'll also notice the absence of snacks on certain days. This is done to give your digestive system a break from constantly digesting food. Your body will be able to spend more energy on breaking down immune complexes within your body and restoring greater health. Finally, you'll notice that the lighter "cleanse" days are only every other day during this week.

Monday

Breakfast Fresh Pressed Green Juice (your choice)

Snack n/a

Lunch Kale Salad

Snack n/a

Dinner Quinoa Tabouli

Tuesday

Breakfast Fresh Pressed Green Juice (your choice)

Snack ½ handful almonds, walnuts, pumpkin seeds

Lunch Mock Tuna Salad

Snack Coconut Chocolate Truffles (2 or 3)

Dinner Waldorf Salad

Wednesday

Breakfast   Fresh Pressed Green Juice (your choice)

Snack   Spirulina (mixed with water or juice)

Lunch   Green Soup

Snack   n/a

Dinner   Smoothie (your choice)

Thursday

Breakfast   Fresh Pressed Green Juice (your choice)

Snack   Fruit of choice with Almond Butter

Lunch   Nori Wrap with Mango Chutney

Snack   Corn and Lentil Salad

Dinner   Veggie Sushi

Friday

Breakfast   Fresh Pressed Green Juice (your choice)

Snack   n/a

Lunch   Smoothie (your choice)

Snack   n/a

Dinner   Everything in the Fridge Salad

Week 5

<u>**Monday**</u>

Breakfast	Morning Muesli
Snack	Small handful goji berries and raw cacao nibs
Lunch	Green Beans and Brown Rice in Curry Sauce
Snack	Fresh Pressed Green Juice (your choice)
Dinner	Wilted Kale Salad

<u>**Tuesday**</u>

Breakfast	Fresh Pressed Green Juice (your choice)
Snack	Fruit (your choice) with ¼ handful almonds, pumpkin seeds
Lunch	Smoothie (your choice)
Snack	Mexican Salad
Dinner	Banana and Strawberry Cream Pie

<u>**Wednesday**</u>

Breakfast	Coco-Vanilla Porridge
Snack	Spirulina (mixed with water or juice)
Lunch	Quinoa Salad
Snack	Chic pea Hummus with veggies
Dinner	Cal-Mag Soup

Thursday

Breakfast   Smoothie (your choice)

Snack   Celery with Nut Butter and Raisins

Lunch   Watermelon Soup

Snack   Guacamole Salsa with Veggies

Dinner   Zucchini Pasta with Marinara Sauce

Friday

Breakfast   Blueberry Morning

Snack   Fresh Pressed Juice (your choice)

Lunch   Nori Wrap with Olive Tapenade

Snack   ¼ handful walnuts and sunflower seeds

Dinner   Creamy Carrot Ginger Soup

Week 6

Monday

Breakfast   Smoothie (your choice)

Snack   Small handful goji berries and raw cacao nibs

Lunch   Quinoa Paella

Snack   Traditional Guacamole with veggies

Dinner   Everything in the Fridge Salad

Tuesday

Breakfast   Fresh Pressed Green Juice (your choice)

Snack   Fruit (your choice) with ¼ handful almonds, pumpkin seeds

Lunch   Popeye's Herb and Spinach Soup

Snack   Celery with Nut Butter and Raisins

Dinner   Veggie Sushi with Spicy Mayonnaise

Wednesday

Breakfast   Blueberry Morning

Snack   Spirulina (mixed with water or juice)

Lunch   Collard Taco with Tomato Salsa & Mango and Avocado Salad

Snack   Chic pea Hummus with veggies

Dinner   Smoothie (your choice)

Thursday

Breakfast	Fresh Pressed Green Juice (your choice)
Snack	¼ handful almonds, pumpkin seeds
Lunch	Curry Kale Salad
Snack	Fresh Pressed Juice (your choice)
Dinner	Sweet Potato Pasta with Pesto Sauce

Friday

Breakfast	Porridge of Champions
Snack	Fresh Pressed Juice (your choice)
Lunch	A Date with Kale & Marinated Broccoli
Snack	Sunset Pudding
Dinner	Salad Slaw

Week 7

Monday

Breakfast   Fresh Pressed Green Juice (your choice)

Snack   Small handful goji berries and raw cacao nibs

Lunch   Collard Taco with Tomato Salsa

Snack   Strawberry – Banana Gelato

Dinner   Yammy's Pad Thai

Tuesday

Breakfast   Raw Oatmeal

Snack   Fruit (your choice) with ¼ handful almonds, pumpkin seeds

Lunch   Red Pepper Cream Soup

Snack   Fresh Pressed Green Juice (your choice)

Dinner   Sweet Potato Pasta with Marinara Sauce

Wednesday

Breakfast   Smoothie (your choice)

Snack   Spirulina (mixed with water or juice)

Lunch   Salad from the Sea

Snack   Lentil Hummus with veggies

Dinner   Veggie Sushi with Spicy Mayonnaise

Thursday

Breakfast   Fresh Pressed Green Juice (your choice)

Snack   ¼ handful almonds, pumpkin seeds

Lunch   Wilted Kale Salad

Snack   Smoothie (your choice)

Dinner   Quinoa Paella with Olive Tapenade

Friday

Breakfast   Porridge of Champions

Snack   Fresh Pressed Juice (your choice)

Lunch   A Date with Kale & Marinated Broccoli

Snack   Orange Coconut Fudge (1 bar)

Dinner   Cream of Tomato Soup

Week 8

Week 8 marks the beginning of another mild cleansing week. Incorporating more green smoothies and juices while limiting the total amount of foods consumed will heighten your body's energy and further cleanse your system. The body is an amazing machine and will naturally cleanse and heal itself if we would just let it! Unfortunately, most of the time we pollute it with too much food and too many non-foods that are not nearly as nourishing as they should be. The 2 liquid days this week will allow your body to better heal itself by imposing less stress on the digestive system yet still providing vital nutrients for repair and rejuvenation. If you feel any detoxification symptoms such as headaches or skin outbreaks, drink plenty of water to help flush out the newly released toxins. These are simply signs that your body is ridding itself of waste that has built up over many years of abuse. In general, the more toxic you are, the greater the intensity of detoxification symptoms you will experience. Everyone is different, but more often than not these symptoms will start to disappear within a few days and you will be cleaner, healthier, and more energetic than ever!

Monday – liquid day

Breakfast   Fresh Pressed Green Juice (your choice)

Snack   n/a

Lunch   Smoothie (your choice)

Snack   n/a

Dinner   Fresh Pressed Green Juice (your choice)

Tuesday

Breakfast   Raw Oatmeal

Snack   Fruit (your choice) with ¼ handful almonds, pumpkin seeds

Lunch   Nori Wrap with Mango Chutney

Snack   Fresh Pressed Green Juice (your choice)

Dinner   Mango and Avocado Salad

Wednesday

Breakfast   Smoothie (your choice)

Snack   Spirulina (mixed with water or juice)

Lunch   Corn and Lentil Salad

Snack   Fresh Pressed Juice(your choice)

Dinner   Quinoa Tabouli & Marinated Broccoli

Thursday

Breakfast   Fresh Pressed Green Juice (your choice)

Snack   ¼ handful almonds, pumpkin seeds

Lunch   Wilted Kale Salad

Snack   Smoothie (your choice)

Dinner   Quinoa Paella with Olive Tapenade

Friday – liquid day

Breakfast   Fresh Pressed Juice (your choice)

Snack   n/a

Lunch   Fresh Pressed Green Juice (your choice)

Snack   n/a

Dinner   Smoothie (your choice)

Week 9

<u>Monday</u>

Breakfast   Fresh Pressed Green Juice (your choice)

Snack   Chic Pea Hummus with veggies

Lunch   Waldorf Salad

Snack   Smoothie (your choice)

Dinner   Veggie Sushi with Spicy Mayonnaise

<u>Tuesday</u>

Breakfast   Coco-Vanilla Porridge

Snack   Spirulina (mixed with water or juice)

Lunch   Alkalizing Cucumber Soup

Snack   Fresh Pressed Green Juice (your choice)

Dinner   Zucchini Pasta with Pesto Sauce

<u>Wednesday</u>

Breakfast   Smoothie (your choice)

Snack   ¼ handful almonds, walnuts, pumpkin/sunflower seeds

Lunch   Sweet Apple Nori Wrap

Snack   Celery with Nut Butter and Raisins

Dinner   Collard Rolls

Thursday

Breakfast   Bananas, Berries, and Cream

Snack   Spirulina (mixed with water or juice)

Lunch   Salad from the Sea

Snack   Fresh Pressed Juice (your choice)

Dinner   Quinoa Tabouli with Mashed Potatoes

Friday

Breakfast   Fresh Pressed Green Juice (your choice)

Snack   Fruit (your choice) with Nut Butter

Lunch   Kale Salad

Snack   Pistachio Halvah

Dinner   Sweet Apple Nori Wrap

Week 10

<u>Monday</u>

Breakfast   Fresh Pressed Green Juice (your choice)

Snack   Chic Pea Hummus with veggies

Lunch   Wilted Kale Salad

Snack   Marinated Broccoli

Dinner   Smoothie (your choice)

<u>Tuesday</u>

Breakfast   Fresh Pressed Green Juice (your choice)

Snack   Spirulina (mixed with water or juice)

Lunch   Waldorf Salad and Olive Tapenade

Snack   Smoothie (your choice)

Dinner   Everything in the Fridge Salad

<u>Wednesday</u>

Breakfast   Fresh Pressed Green Juice (your choice)

Snack   ¼ handful almonds, walnuts, pumpkin/sunflower seeds

Lunch   Sweet Apple Nori Wrap

Snack   ¼ handful goji berries and cacao nibs

Dinner   Collard Taco with Tomato Salsa

Thursday

Breakfast   Fresh Pressed Green Juice (your choice)

Snack   Spirulina (mixed with water or juice)

Lunch   Avocado and Mango Salad

Snack   Lentil Hummus with veggies

Dinner   Quinoa Salad

Friday

Breakfast   Fresh Pressed Green Juice (your choice)

Snack   Fruit (your choice) with Nut Butter

Lunch   Curry Kale Salad

Snack   Smoothie (your choice)

Dinner   Arugula Salad

Week 11

Monday

Breakfast   Fresh Pressed Green Juice (your choice)

Snack   Fruit with Nut Butter

Lunch   Everything in the Fridge Salad

Snack   Marinated Broccoli

Dinner   Raspberry Cheesecake

Tuesday

Breakfast   Fresh Pressed Green Juice (your choice)

Snack   Spirulina (mixed with water or juice)

Lunch   Collard Taco with Tomato Salsa

Snack   Smoothie (your choice)

Dinner   Quinoa Paella

Wednesday

Breakfast   Fresh Pressed Green Juice (your choice)

Snack   ¼ handful almonds, walnuts, pumpkin/sunflower seeds

Lunch   Smoothie (your choice)

Snack   ¼ handful goji berries and cacao nibs

Dinner   Mock Tuna Salad

Thursday

Breakfast   Fresh Pressed Green Juice (your choice)

Snack   Fruit (your choice) with ¼ cup almonds, walnuts, seeds

Lunch   Broccoli Soup

Snack   Lentil Hummus with veggies

Dinner   Veggie Sushi with Spicy Mayonnaise

Friday

Breakfast   Fresh Pressed Green Juice (your choice)

Snack   Celery with Nut Butter and Raisins

Lunch   Pineapple – Cucumber Gazpacho

Snack   Spirulina (mixed with water or juice)

Dinner   Salad from the Sea

Week 12

By now you will have experienced 2 weeks of mild cleansing (Weeks 4 and 8). This Week 12 menu will act as your 3rd and final cleansing week. Because you've progressed to incorporate more raw foods into your lifestyle your body will have transformed already. However, this week will feature 2 days of Master Cleansing to further jump start your body's ability to detoxify and purify itself. The **Master Cleanser** is simply a concoction of water, maple syrup, fresh lemon juice, and ground cayenne pepper. Throughout these 2 days the goal is to eat or drink nothing but this Master Cleanser or water (see rules below).

By no means are you obligated to follow this 2-day Master Cleanse but if you feel like you can and want to explore it, then please do. I would also recommend that you limit your physical activity during these 2 days as your body will be low in fuel. Upon completing the 2-day fast you will reintroduce nutrients into your body via juices and slowly progress back into solid foods (simply follow the Meal Plan). It is wise to make a gradual transition back into a regular diet, rather than just going out for dinner after a few days of fasting. Your digestion has been at rest, so you need to focus on chewing your foods really well. Papaya and pineapple are also incorporated after your 2-day cleanse as they contain natural digestive enzymes papain and bromelain, respectively, which help to restore proper digestive function.

Here is the recipe for the **Master Cleanser**:
- 2 tbsp fresh lemon juice
- 1-2 tbsp pure maple syrup
- ½ tsp ground cayenne pepper
- 8 ounces spring water

Rules of the Master Cleanse:
- Drink 8 to 12 glasses of the Master Cleanser throughout the day.
- Eat or drink nothing else except water or peppermint/chamomile herbal tea.

Monday – Master Cleanse Day #1

Drink 8 to 12 glasses of the Master Cleanser and water throughout the day.

Tuesday – Master Cleanse Day #2

Drink 8 to 12 glasses of the Master Cleanser and water throughout the day.

Wednesday

Breakfast   Fresh Pressed Green Juice (your choice)

Snack   Papaya or Pineapple

Lunch   Fresh Pressed Juice (your choice)

Snack   Papaya or Pineapple

Dinner   Fresh Pressed Juice (your choice)

Thursday

Breakfast   Smoothie (your choice)

Snack   Papaya or Pineapple

Lunch   Creamy Carrot Ginger Soup

Snack   Fresh Pressed Green Juice (your choice)

Dinner   Creamy Tomato Soup

Friday

Breakfast   Fresh Pressed Green Juice (your choice)

Snack   Bananas, Berries, and Cream

Lunch   Pineapple – Cucumber Gazpacho

Snack   Spirulina (mixed with water or juice)

Dinner   Cal-Mag Soup and Quinoa Salad

Healthy
recipe GUIDE

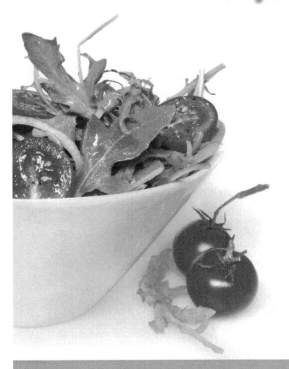

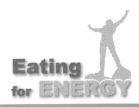

Eating
for ENERGY

Breakfast Cereals

Most store-bought packaged cereals are processed and packaged with ingredients that should not be entering your body. However, there are "commercial" cereals that are better than others.

This section will show you some great tasting and easy to prepare natural healthy cereals that can be enjoyed at anytime of the day. Simply add your favourite Nut Milk (see Smoothie and Juice Guide) and enjoy!

See the **Smoothie and Juice Guide** for more breakfast ideas. Who said breakfast had to be solid?

If you want more recipes...

Then, visit my blog for all our new and delicious concoctions...

http://blog.totalwellnessconsulting.ca

Blueberry Morning

Serves 1 to 2

½ cup fresh blueberries

1 banana, chopped (optional)

½ cup soaked/sprouted buckwheat (optional)

Combine with Nut milk:

¼ cup almonds, presoaked

2 tbsp ground sesame seeds

1 tbsp ground flaxseed

2-3 dates

1-2 tbsp agave nectar

1. For nut milk, blend all ingredients in a high speed blender until smooth and creamy.
2. Pour over blueberries and serve.

Porridge of Champions

Serves 1 to 2

½ cup buckwheat groats, sprouted

½ cup raisins

½ cup goji berries (optional)

½ cup dried apricots, diced

½ cup hemp seeds

½ cup pumpkin seeds

½ cup sunflower seeds

½ cup chopped almonds

1. Soak ingredients overnight in nut milk of choice.
2. **Top with**: ground sesame seeds, ground flax seeds, and agave nectar.

Morning Muesli

Serves 1 to 2

2 cups of nuts (your choice), chopped

1 cup berries (your choice)

1 apple, diced

1 banana, sliced

2 tbsp dried shredded coconut

1 tbsp ground sesame seeds

1 tbsp ground flaxseed

1-2 cups *Nut Milk*

1. Mix together all the nuts, berries, and fruit in a bowl.
2. Top with shredded coconut flakes, and ground sesame and flaxseeds.
3. Pour your favourite *Nut Milk* over top and enjoy!

Coco - Vanilla Porridge

Serves 4 to 6

2 cups almonds, soaked overnight

2 cups young coconut meat

1½ cups young coconut water

2 tbsp vanilla extract

1 tbsp raw coconut butter

1 tbsp agave nectar

1. Combine all ingredients in a high speed blender and process until smooth and creamy.

Raw Oatmeal

Serves 1 to 2

2 cups oat groats, sprouted

½ cup blueberries (and/or any other fruit)

2 tbsp ground flaxseed

3 tbsp raisins, soaked

2-3 tbsp sunflower seeds

1-2 cups Nut Milk recipe of your choice

1. Sprout oat groats following Soaking/Sprouting 101.
2. Combine all ingredients in a bowl.
3. Pour Nut Milk over top and enjoy.

Bananas, Berries, and Cream

Serves 2

2 bananas

1 cup blueberries

1-2 tbsp ground flaxseeds

¾ cup almonds, soaked

1½ cups cashews

2 cups fresh pineapple chunks

1. In a food processor, grind the almonds into a fine powder and then add in cashews and pineapple chunks. This is your pineapple nut cream OR milk.
2. Pour the pineapple nut cream over the fruit and and enjoy!
3. Top with ground flaxseeds.

Soups

Slightly different from their conventional piping hot counterparts, these refreshing and quick to prepare soups are wonderfully tasty and nutritious.

I love using them during warmer times of the year. And because they aren't heated, they maintain their inherit wholeness, energy, and enzyme-rich properties. Since they maintain their life force, they are best consumed immediately after preparing but if you absolutely must, they should be ok to keep in the refrigerator for up to 24 hours.

All you need to prepare them is a blender (or food processor).

Creamy Carrot Ginger Soup

I absolutely love this soup. The ginger gives it a little kick and its creaminess is so satisfying. *Serves 1 to 2*

3 cups fresh carrot juice
1 small, ripe avocado (pit and skin removed)
½ cup coconut meat (optional)
½ cup lime juice
2 tbsp agave nectar
1 tbsp minced ginger
¼ tsp cayenne
¼ tsp sea salt
Few sprigs of cilantro for garnish (optional)

1. In a high-speed blender, puree all ingredients until completely smooth. Taste for seasoning and add garnish is desired.

Popeye's Spinach & Herb Soup

Eat this enough and you'll be strong like popeye!

Serves 2 to 4

3 cups fresh raw spinach

1 cup sweet peas

3 cups almond milk

1 kiwi, peeled

2 celery stalks

½ handful cilantro

4 basil leaves

2 green onions, diced

Juice of 1 lime

Pinch of sea salt or kelp/dulse flakes

1. Place all ingredients in a high-powered blender and process until smooth.

Red Pepper Cream Soup

Serves 2 to 3

1 avocado (pit and skin removed)

1 red bell pepper, chopped

2 cups water or almond milk

½ handful of cilantro, chopped

½ tsp of dulse flakes

pinch of oregano

1. Blend all ingredients in a blender or food processor.

Pineapple-Cucumber Gazpacho

This is a wonderful dish to serve on a warm summer's day. If you like heat add in the jalapeno.

Serves 2 to 4

2 cups chopped peeled cucumber

2 cups chopped fresh pineapple

½ cup fresh pineapple juice

½ green onion, chopped

½ jalapeno (optional)

½ tbsp lime juice

½ handful cilantro leaves

2 tbsp olive oil

½ handful finely chopped macadamia nuts

1. In a blender, add 1 ½ cups each of cucumber and pineapple, the pineapple juice, green onion, jalapeno (if desired), lime juice, and a pinch of sea salt. Blend until smooth.
2. Add the remaining ½ cup of pineapple and cucumber, the cilantro, and 1 tbsp of olive oil. Pulse the blender a few times – the gazpacho should remain chunky. Place in refrigerator to cool if desired.
3. Add macadamia nuts before serving, and drizzle remaining olive oil.

Broccoli Soup

If you don't like broccoli – you're about to start. This is a wonderful way to enjoy the cancer-fighting powers that broccoli possesses. Again, the creaminess and smooth texture make it wonderfully palatable. Recipe inspired by Alissa Cohen's *Living on Live Food* (great book!)[38]

Serves 1 to 2

3 cups almond milk
2 cups chopped broccoli
1 avocado
½ clove of garlic
1 tbsp olive oil
1 tsp sea salt (or dulse/kelp flakes)
½ tsp ground cumin
pinch of black pepper

1. Blend all ingredients in a blender until creamy.

---

[38] Cohen, A. (2004). *Living on Live Food*. Cohen Publishing Company. Kittery, Maine, USA.

Alkalizing Cucumber Soup

Cucumber has a neutralizing effect on our body and provides great alkalinity. This is a wonderful soup for anyone with indigestion.

Serves 1 to 2

1 avocado

1 cucumber, chopped

4 tbsp dill weed or chopped fresh dill

2 tsp lemon juice

½ tsp sea salt or kelp/dulse flakes

1. Blend all ingredients in a blender until smooth and creamy.

Watermelon Soup

Serves 2 to 3

5 cups watermelon, seeded and cubed

2 cups mango, peeled and diced

¼ cup lime juice

3 tbsp fresh mint, chopped

1 tbsp fresh ginger, minced

1 tbsp agave nectar

pinch of ground cardamom

1. Place 3 ½ cups watermelon and 1 cup mango in a food processor or blender and blend until smooth.
2. Dice up the remaining watermelon and mango into tiny pieces and add to the puree.
3. In a small separate bowl, combine lime juice, mint, ginger, agave nectar and cardamom. Add this to the previous mixture and stir well.
4. Chill and serve.

Cal-Mag Soup

This soup doesn't need an explanation – just look at the ingredients!

Serves 2 to 4

10 kale leaves, chopped

1 handful parsley

2 cloves garlic, chopped

¼ red onion, chopped

2 lemons, outer skin removed

1 avocado

1 tomato

2 yellow bell peppers

½ cup pumpkin seeds

¼ cup ground sesame seeds

½ cup of dulse strips/flakes

1 tsp of sea salt

3 tbsp flax oil

Add water as needed to get proper consistency

1. Blend all ingredients in a blender until smooth

Green Soup

Serves 2

Most of us are way too acidic due to our unbalanced diets. This soup is highly alkalizing. The avocado provides healthy fats, as well as a cream-like consistency.

1 avocado
1 red pepper
1 cucumber, peeled
2 spring onions
2 ribs celery, chopped
1 cup spinach, packed
¼ cup parsley, packed
1 clove garlic, minced
A pinch of cayenne
Braggs liquid aminos to taste
Juice of 1 lemon or lime

1. Combine all ingredients in a food processor until creamy and smooth.

Cream of Tomato Soup

Serves 2

¼ cup diced onion

1 clove garlic

4 stalks celery

2 carrots

½ cup basil

4 tomatoes

1 cup water

½ cup cashews, soaked

4 dates, soaked

A pinch of cayenne and Braggs to taste

1. Combine all ingredients in a food processor until creamy and smooth.

Sandwiches and Wraps

Put away the bread and bagels. Get ready for some great tasting, nourishing, and energizing sandwiches and wraps that require no bread or wheat whatsoever. For these quick and easy recipes you'll be using the leaves of leafy green vegetables or nori as the base of your sandwich/wrap.

Many of these can be prepared ahead of time and taken to work. Feel free to experiment and add some of the sauces/dips outlined in the Dressings, Dips, and Sauces section to create a different flavour for any of the following sandwiches/wraps.

Nori Wrap

This is one of my all-time favourite wraps. It's so easy to prepare and it's packed full of nutrients and great taste. For even greater taste, add any one of the dips, sauces, or dressings.
Makes 6 wraps (1-2 servings)

6 sheets of Nori
1 avocado, thinly sliced
1 mango, thinly sliced
1 cup alfalfa sprouts
¼ cucumber, thinly sliced
½ sprouted grain/legume of choice (optional)
4 radishes, sliced (optional)

1. Lay out 1 sheet of Nori and place within it a desired amount of each ingredient.
2. Roll Nori (with ingredients inside) up into a wrap and enjoy.
3. You can also use any of the sauces, dips, or dressings (described later) for added flavour.

Sweet Apple Nori Wrap

Inspired by Alissa Cohen's *Living on Live Food*.

Makes 2 wraps (1-2 servings)

2 sheets of Nori
1 avocado, thinly sliced
1 apple, thinly sliced
1-2 tbsp agave nectar
1 cup chopped lettuce

1. Lay out each sheet of Nori and place within it a desired amount of apple and avocado.
2. Pour agave over top the avocado and apple, then place a small amount of lettuce over top.
3. Roll nori together and enjoy!

A Date with Kale

This has quickly become one of my most enjoyable meals. It's so simple, tastes great, and is packed full of nutrients. Inspired by David Wolfe!

Serves 1 to 2

10 kale leaves
10 dates, pitted
1 avocado
1 mango (optional)

1. Cut the avocado (and mango) into 10 pieces.
2. Place a date with an avocado slice inside a kale leaf and wrap like a burrito.

Collard Taco with Tomato Salsa

Ground walnuts give a texture of real taco meat. Combined with the Mexican spices and Tomato Salsa, this "taco" will put other ones to shame.

Serves 3 to 4

2 cups walnuts, ground in a food processor

1 tbsp ground cumin

1 tbsp ground coriander

3 to 4 collard green leaves

1 cup shredded romaine lettuce

1 recipe Tomato Salsa

1. In a food processor, pulse walnuts until they look like "meaty"
2. In a bowl, combine the walnuts, cumin, and coriander, and mix well.
3. Spread ¼ of the walnut mixture along the center stem of each collard green leaf, then add a layer of shredded lettuce. Top with ¼ cup of the salsa and enjoy!

Collard Rolls

Recipe inspired by Alissa Cohen's *Living on Live Food.*
Makes 2 large wraps (1-2 servings)

2 large collard leaves
1 zucchini, shredded
1 carrot, shredded
1 avocado or 1 recipe Traditional Guacamole
½ onion, sliced into ringlets
1 cup Portobello mushrooms, cut into bite size pieces
2 cups chopped lettuce
1 cup Bragg Liquid Aminos or Tamari

1. Marinate the onions and mushrooms in Bragg's or Tamari for at least 10 minutes. Then drain well.
2. Lay the collard leaves flat with the inside facing up.
3. Place desired amount of ingredients inside the collard leaves and add in the onion and mushroom mixture.
4. Roll leaf up and enjoy!

Salads

Salads are great! Salads taste delicious and are tremendously nutritious. If you're tired of the same old boring salad, then just wait until you give these a whirl. They are packed full of high quality ingredients and will leave you feeling satiated and energized. Remember Success Habit #1? Eat one big green salad every day. Salads should truly be the foundation of your diet, especially if you're looking to lose weight. If you don't want to lose weight, then salads should still be a major part of your diet for they can provide substantial amounts of calories (depending on which ingredients are used) while meeting peak nutrition standards.

Kale Salad

Serves 1 to 2

2 small or 1 large bunch of Kale
2 tbsp olive oil
2 tbsp lemon juice
1 tsp chili powder
pinch of sea salt

1. Clean kale. Tear or cut into small pieces.
2. Add all ingredients in a bowl and mix

Curry Kale Salad

Serves 1 to 2

Dressing
3 tbsp olive oil
Juice of ½ lemon
1 ½ tsp fresh curry powder
1 tsp cayenne powder
2 cloves fresh garlic, minced
1 tsp fresh ginger, grated
2-4 dates, soaked

1. Blend everything in a high-speed blender. Add water to thin it out if needed.
2. Keep refrigerated until ready to use.

Salad
1 bunch kale

1. Get the kale, roll it up and chop it into thin strips. Place the kale in a salad bowl and dress up the salad with as much dressing, as you like.

Waldorf Salad

Serves 1 to 2

2 apples, chopped (fuji)

2 tomatoes, chopped

2 avocados, chopped

1 orange or yellow sweet pepper, chopped

1/2 sweet onion or shallot, chopped

handful sprouts (alfalfa, radish, etc)

2 tbsp olive oil

pinch of sea salt

dash of cayenne pepper and onion powder

1. Combine all ingredients in a salad bowl

Thai Salad

Serves 4 to 6

4 cucumbers
Juice of 1 lemon
1 bunch dill, finely chopped
1 bunch cilantro, finely chopped
1 medium sized onion, diced
3 tsp hot curry powder
1 tsp sea salt
3 tbsp agave nectar or honey
2 tbsp olive oil
1 cup soaked sunflower seeds

1. Peel and slice the cucumbers into thin circles and transfer to a bowl.
2. Next, finely chop the cilantro and dill and mix with the cucumbers.
3. Add the onion, lemon juice, and the olive oil.
4. Finish by adding the rest of the ingredients and mixing well.

Everything in the Fridge Salad

This salad (like many others) just about throws in the kitchen sink there's so much in it!

Serves 2 to 4

4 cups organic greens

1 or 2 fennel bulbs, chopped

1 red onion, diced

1 clove of garlic. minced

1 red pepper, diced

1 orange pepper, diced

4 tomatoes

½ cup pumpkin sprouts or seeds, soaked

3 stalks of celery, chopped

2 avocados, peeled and stoned

10 macadamia nuts, chopped

10 olives, pitted

1 cup of watercress

4 dates, stoned

1 cup arame, soaked

1. Combine all ingredients in a large salad bowl.
2. Add any of the dressings, give it a toss, and enjoy.

Arugula Salad

Serves 2 to 4

For the dressing:
4 lemons, peeled and quartered (leave some of the white pith)
2 tbsp raw honey
3 tbsp olive oil
Pinch of sea salt

1. Blend all ingredients in a high speed blender – makes about 1 cup.

For the salad:
4 cups arugula leaves
1 pear, cut into shavings with a peeler
½ cup dried cherries or cranberries
½ cup pumpkin seeds

1. Toss ingredients in a salad bowl and mix in dressing.

Salad from the Sea

Serves 2 to 4

For the dressing:
½ cup white miso
3 tbsp agave nectar
¼ cup sesame oil
Juice of 1 lemon
2 tbsp minced ginger

1. In a blender, process all ingredients until smooth – makes about 2 cups.

For the salad:
¼ cup dried wakame, lightly soaked
¼ cup dried hijiki, lightly soaked
¼ cup dried arame, lightly soaked
½ sheet dried nori, cut into thin strips
1 cucumber, peeled and julienned
2 beets, peeled and julienned
1 radish, peeled and julienned
1 green onion, thinly sliced
1 tbsp white sesame seeds

1. Soak the sea vegetables until soft (but not waterlogged). This should take about 5-10 minutes.
2. Drain the sea vegetables with your hands squeezing out as much water as possible.
3. Add all ingredients into a large bowl
4. Add the dressing and serve

Mango and Avocado Salad

Serves 2

4 cups mixed greens

1 avocado

1 mango

¼ cup red onion

1. Toss ingredients in a salad bowl and mix in **Simple Vinaigrette** dressing.

Carrot Salad

Serves 1 to 2

4 carrots, spiralized or grated in food processor

½ cup raisins, soaked

½ cup walnuts, chopped

1 tsp cinnamon

1. Toss ingredients in a salad bowl and mix in **Simple Vinaigrette** dressing.

Mexican Salad

Serves 2

2 corn on the cob
1 tomato, cubed
1 avocado, cubed
1 red pepper, cubed
½ cucumber, cubed

1. De-cob corn using a knife, chop up additional ingredients bite size and add to a medium bowl.
2. Top with dressing of choice (I like the Simple Vinaigrette).

Salad Slaw

Say goodbye to your traditional slaw made with mayonnaise! This version is way healthier, and has replaced the unhealthy heated, trans-fat, canola oil, based mayonnaise with a raw healthy fat to keep the cell walls in your body flaccid for membrane transport. The sauerkraut provides the body with healthy bacteria.
Serves 2

2 large handfuls mixed greens

4 carrots

3 radishes

¼ cup red onion

1 orange, juiced

½ avocado

2 heaping forkfuls of fermented sauerkraut (found refrigerated in health food stores)

1. Place mixed greens in a large bowl
2. Roughly chop the carrots, radishes, and red onion and place in food processor. Process until finely shredded and empty onto the greens.
3. Roughly chop the avocado and place in food processor (no need to clean it from previous use) with orange juice and process until creamy. Pour onto Salad mixture and mix by hand.
4. Heap sauerkraut on top and serve.

Corn and Lentil Salad

Serves 1 to 2

1 cup sprouted lentils
1 tbsp olive oil
3 cups fresh corn kernels, (5 or 6 ears)
½ cup red onion
cayenne to taste
½ cup cilantro, chopped

1. Using a knife, skin the corn kernels off each cob/ear.
2. Add with all other ingredients in a salad bowl and apply dressing (below).

Dressing: Process the following in a food processor until smooth:1 tomato, 2 tbsp olive oil, 2 dates (soaked), ½ clove garlic (minced) 1 lemon or lime (juiced) or 1 tbsp apple cider vinegar

Wilted Kale Salad

This salad will absolutely blow your mind. I couldn't believe how good it was the first time I had it!

Serves 2

1 head kale

2 tsp sea salt

2 tomatoes, chopped

1 tbsp sesame seeds

1 tbsp hemp seeds

½ of an avocado

1 lemon, juiced

1 tbsp Braggs liquid aminos

1 tbsp olive oil or flax oil

1 clove garlic

1 tsp cumin

½ tsp ground red pepper flakes (or to taste)

1. Wash kale, remove leaves from stems, and chop finely.
2. Sprinkle kale with sea salt and work salt into the leaves until they appear to be "cooked." You will know when it's ready because you will be able to squeeze liquid out of the mixture. Squeeze the salty liquid out and discard.
3. Add tomatoes, hemp seeds, and sesame seeds to the kale and mix.
4. **For the dressing**: smash up avocado with a knife or fork and place it in a food processor with the lemon juice, Braggs, oil, garlic clove, cumin, and red pepper flakes. Process until it resembles mayonnaise, and mix into the kale mixture.

Dressings, Dips, and Sauces

Sesame Avocado Dressing

Serves 1 to 2

1 cup soaked sesame seeds (overnight or 4 hours)

2 small avocados

½ cup apple cider vinegar

12 mejool dates, soaked

1 cup water

1 tsp sea salt

    1. Blend all ingredients in a blender or food processor

Simple Vinaigrette

Makes ¼ cup

2-3 tbsp olive oil

1 tbsp apple cider vinegar

Juice of ½ lemon

Pinch of ground black pepper

Pinch of sea salt

    1. Using a fork, whisk all ingredients in a cup and pour over salad.

Sun-Dried Tomato Dressing

1 tomato

1/3 cup diced onion

1 clove garlic, minced

2 tbsp olive oil

1 tbsp balsamic vinegar

½ cup sun-dried tomatoes

½ cup basil

2 dates, soaked

1. Combine all ingredients in a food processor and blend until smooth and semi-liquid.

Tahini Fig Dressing

4 ripe figs

3 tbsp tahini (ground sesame seeds)

2 tbsp agave nectar

1 tbsp apple cider vinegar

1. Combine all ingredients in a food processor and blend until smooth and semi-liquid.

Raspberry Orange Vinaigrette

½ cup fresh orange juice (2 oranges)

½ cup raspberries

1 tsp orange zest

1 tsp minced shallot

1 tbsp apple cider vinegar

1 tbsp olive oil

1. Using a citrus juicer, juice both oranges
2. Combine all ingredients in a food processor and blend until smooth and semi-liquid.

Garlic Dill Dressing

Serves 1 to 2

1 cup cashews, soaked

1 cup water

1 oz fresh dill

1 oz fresh chives

2 cloves garlic

1 tsp salt

1. Blend all ingredients in a blender or food processor

Guacamole Salsa

Serves 1 to 2

1 avocado, diced

1 tbsp minced red onion

4 tbsp chopped fresh herbs (parsley, cilantro, marjoram)

1 tbsp lemon or lime juice

½ clove minced garlic

1 tsp cayenne powder

1-2 pinch Celtic sea salt

1. Combine everything together and put the avocado pit in the mixture to prevent oxidation.

Traditional Guacamole

Serves 4

4 ripe avocados

2 roma tomatoes, diced fine

½ red onion, minced

½ handful cilantro, minced

1-2 cloves garlic, minced

Juice of 1 lime

Pinch of sea salt

1/2 - 1 jalapeno, seeded and minced fine (optional)

1. Place all ingredients in a bowl with a flat bottom and mash it with a potato masher. Stir well and keep refrigerated. This dish will brown on the areas exposed to air within a few hours, so serve it shortly after making it or just stir again before serving.

Creamy Cucumber Dressing/Dip

This is a divine dressing and makes a delicious dip for parties or anytime. This is just wonderful served over a bed of fresh spinach leaves with tomatoes and orange segments, or you use it as a dip with fresh veggies.

Serves 8-10 as a dip, or keep on hand to use in salads

1 cucumber, peeled and cut into large pieces

1 avocado

handful chopped cilantro

1-2 green onions

3-4 basil fresh leaves, chopped

2 tbsp flaxseed oil

1 tbsp olive oil

2 tbsp agave nectar

2 tsp apple cider vinegar

Pinch of sea salt

1 tsp fresh dill

1. Place all ingredients in a blender or food processor. Blend until completely smooth and creamy.

Mango Chutney

Serves 2 to 4

2 mangos
½ lime juiced
2 tbsp minced ginger
2 green onions. diced
½ small jalapeno, cored and seeded, diced
Pinch of sea salt
Small handful cilantro leaves

1. Place all ingredients in food processor and pulse to combine well, but keep it chunky. Store in a covered container in the refrigerator for up to 3 days.

Olive Tapenade

Serves 2 to 4

3 cups pitted kalamata olives
½ cup olive oil
Juice of ¼ lemon
1 small handful of parsley
½ cup sun-dried tomatoes (optional)
Freshly ground black pepper
Pinch of sea salt

1. Process the olives in a food processor.
2. With the motor running add the olive oil and lemon juice and process until smooth.
3. Add the parsley and process to combine
4. Store in a covered container in the refrigerator for up to 1 week.

Garlic Mayonnaise

1 avocado
½ orange juiced
1 clove garlic, minced

1. Juice orange using a citrus juicer
2. Blend all ingredients in a food processor until smooth

Marinara Sauce

This is a wonderful sauce for pasta and is even great when used as a dip.

Serves 2 to 4

4 cloves garlic, diced
1 red bell pepper (optional)
1 cup sun dried tomato, soaked
3 cups chopped tomatoes
4 dates, pitted and soaked
¼ red onion, diced
2 tbsp olive oil
½ handful parsley, chopped
½ handful basil
1/3 cup olives, pitted (optional)
Pinch of sea salt or kelp/dulse flakes

1. In a food processor, pulse all ingredients until smooth.

Spicy Mayonnaise

This is a great sauce to use with the Sushi rolls.

1 avocado
Juice of ½ orange
¼ tsp crushed red pepper flakes
2 tbsp onion, minced
1 tbsp flax oil
1 tsp ginger, minced

1. Juice orange using a citrus juicer
2. Blend all ingredients in a food processor until smooth

Pesto Sauce

Add this delicious sauce to your favourite raw pasta. Absolutely delicious!
Serves 2 to 4

3 cups basil leaves
1-2 cloves garlic, minced
½ cup pine nuts
¼ cup water
1/3 cup nutritional yeast flakes
Juice of ¼ lemon
½ cup olive oil

1. In a food processor, pulse all ingredients until smooth.

Hummus

This is a great dip for your favourite veggies. High in calcium, protein, and great in taste.

Makes about 4 cups

2 cups chickpeas, sprouted (you can even use sprouted lentils instead)
4 cloves garlic, minced
½ cup raw tahini (ground sesame)
Juice of 2 lemons
1 cup parsley, chopped
2-3 tbsp olive oil
Sea salt to taste
Pinch of paprika (for garnish)

1. In a food processor, pulse all ingredients until smooth and creamy.
2. Top with a pinch of paprika and serve.

Tomato Salsa

Serves 2 to 4

2 cups chopped tomatoes
½ cup chopped cilantro
½ cup chopped yellow onions or scallions
Juice of ½ lemon
1 tbsp olive oil
4 cloves garlic, minced
1 tsp ground cumin
1tsp ground coriander
Pinch of cayenne
Pinch of sea salt

1. Combine all ingredients in medium sized bowl, mix well, and serve.

Pastas and Noodle Dishes

Instead of traditional wheat-based or rice noodles, these dishes feature vegetable-based noodles that require no cooking.

They are easy to prepare and taste even better!

All you need is a vegetable peeler or a spiralizer to create your noodles. Because these vegetable-based dishes are raw and uncooked, they are enzyme-rich, nourishing, and don't leave you feeling full and fatigued like most conventional pastas.

The following veggies tend to work best as noodles.
- Zucchini
- Cucumber
- Sweet Potato (or any other root vegetable)

To create your noodles:
1. Peel the skin off the vegetable being used
2. Using a peeler or spiraler, you'll be able to shave thin strips vegetable "noodles" that look like traditional fettuccini or spaghetti noodles.
3. Add your noodles to any of the aforementioned sauces (Marinara, Pesto, etc...)

Yammy's Pad Thai

Serves 2 to 4

Pad Thai Sauce:

1 tbsp tahini

1 tbsp almond butter

1/8 cup cashews

1/4 cup sundried tomatoes, soaked

2 dates, soaked 1 hour

Juice of ½ lime

1-2 garlic cloves

1 tsp fresh ginger, grated

Braggs Amino Acids, to taste

Curry powder, to taste

1. Blend in food processor with some water until you reach desired consistency.
2. Serve on your favorite pasta (ie. zucchini, cucumber).
3. Top with red or yellow pepper, diced and marinated Portobellos (below)

Marinated Portobellos:

1 Portobello mushroom

1 part apple cider vinegar

1 part Braggs Amino Acids

2 tbsp olive oil

1 garlic clove, minced

1 tsp fresh ginger, grated

1 tsp agave nectar or honey

1. Cut the mushroom into bite sized pieces.
2. Put them in a bowl with the other ingredients and mix well.
3. Add to Pad Thai

Fettuccini Cheddar Pasta

This is an awesome dish! The nutritional yeast gives it that distinctive cheddar taste. Serve it on your favourite vegetable-based noodle (I like zucchini) and enjoy!

Serves 2

Cheddar Sauce:

½ **large red bell pepper**

¼ **cup water**

1 cup raw cashews, sunflower seeds, or almonds

1 tbsp tahini

2 tbsp nutritional yeast

1 ½ teaspoon sea salt

¼ **onion, diced OR** ¼ **cup green onions, diced**

1 clove garlic, minced

Juice of ½ **lemon**

1. Blend until creamy. Add more water if it is too thick.
2. Pour over your favourite vegetable-based noodle and enjoy.

Other Mains and Sides

Quinoa Paella

Serves 4

1 red pepper, julienned

1 yellow pepper, julienned

2 white onions, sliced into fine rings

2 cups sprouted quinoa

1 cup chopped young tender asparagus

4 ripe tomatoes, finely chopped

4 sun-dried tomatoes, soaked and finely chopped

5 cloves garlic, crushed

4 stalks celery, juiced

Juice of 2 lemons

4 tbsp olive oil

½ cup kalamata olives, pitted and finely chopped

1 tsp saffron powder

1 tsp paprika

1. Place the peppers, asparagus, onions, and crushed garlic in a wide bowl.
2. Mix the celery and lemon juice with the olive oil and pour it over the chopped vegetables. Let vegetables marinate for several hours, until soft and juicy.
3. Sprout quinoa overnight (as prescribed in Sprouting 101) and rinse well before placing in a serving dish.
4. Pour tomatoes, olives, and marinated vegetables over the quinoa.
5. Add a few tablespoons of the marinade and let stand for a few hours before serving.

Quinoa Salad

This recipe is more than just a salad – that's why it's in this section instead of the salad section. It makes a great side to any dish or it can be enjoyed on its own as an appetizing meal.

Serves 2 to 4

2 cups sprouted quinoa
½ onion, finely diced
½ red (or green or yellow) bell pepper
½ cup diced green olives
½ cup white raisins
¼ cup crushed walnuts
Juice of ½ lemon
2-3 tbsp olive oil
Sea salt and pepper to taste

1. Rinse the quinoa thoroughly in cold water and then sprout following the instructions laid out in Soaking/Sprouting 101.
2. In a larger bowl combine the onion, peppers, walnuts, green olives, and raisins.
3. Mix together lemon juice and olive oil as the vinaigrette and add to the bowl, give it a good mix and ENJOY!

Quinoa Tabouli

Serves 4 to 6

4 cups sprouted quinoa (about 2 cups before sprouting)

4 green onions, thinly sliced

20 mint leaves, minced

1 large tomato, finely sliced

1 cucumber, finely diced

¼ cup parsley, minced

4-6 tbsp olive oil

Juice of 1 lemon

1-2 tbsp of tamari or Braggs Liquid Aminos or pinch of sea salt to taste

1. Mix everything together in a large bowl. Let sit for 1 hour to allow the flavours to combine before serving.

Mashed "Potatoes"

Serves 2 to 4

6 cups chopped cauliflower
¼ cup flaxseed oil
1 tbsp Braggs amino acids to taste
Pinch of sea salt

1. Process cauliflower in a food processor with "S" blade; chop until "grainy".
2. Add other ingredients and gently mix

Mock Tuna Salad (with avocado mayo – see below)

Serves 2 to 4

4 cups almonds, soaked

5 stalks celery, diced

6 green onions, sliced thin

2 tbsp parsley

Juice of 1 lemon

2 dashes cayenne

1 clove garlic, diced

Pinch of sea salt or dulse/kelp flakes

1. Puree Almonds in a food processor until fine.
2. In a medium bowl, combine all ingredients and half of the Avocado Mayo (see below). Enjoy atop a piece of Romaine or Napa cabbage, and a slice of tomato.

Avocado Mayo

1 cup pine nuts

1 large avocado

1 tbsp lemon juice

2 tbsp apple cider vinegar

6 dates, soaked and pitted

1/2 clove garlic, diced

Pinch of sea salt

Marinated Broccoli

Serves 2 to 4

1 head broccoli, stems removed
2 tbsp Braggs
2 cloves garlic, minced
1 tbsp ginger, minced
½ tsp nutmeg
1 tbsp agave nectar
2 tbsp sesame seeds

1. Chop the broccoli into bite size pieces (with the stems removed).
2. In a separate bowl, mix together all other ingredients and then drizzle over the broccoli.

Raw Rice

Makes 2 to 3 cups

3 cups cauliflower
2 handfuls of soaked cashews, walnuts, almonds, or pine nuts
4 tbsp ground sesame seeds
1 tbsp ginger, minced
1 tbsp agave nectar
Juice of ½ lemon

1. Throw all ingredients into a food processor and pulse until it resembles rice.

Veggie Sushi with Spicy Mayonnaise

The first time you make these roll will definitely be a learning experience. However, as you become more comfortable with putting them together you will have the ready to serve in just a few minutes and without the trial and error of a novice. These rolls are absolutely delicious!

Yields 10 – 12 rolls

2 sheets of Nori
1 recipe *Raw Rice* **(above)**
¼ cucumber, julienned
½ red pepper, julienned
2 green onions, julienned
½ cup pea or alfalfa sprouts
1 recipe *Spicy Mayonnaise*
3-4 tbsp Tamari Sauce

To assemble:

1. Cover ½ of the nori sheet with rice and ¼ of the sheet with sprouts.
2. Spread a layer of *Spicy Mayonnaise* on top of ½ the rice layer.
3. Lay your julienned vegetables over the other ½ of the rice layer.
4. Tightly roll using your hands, or a sushi mat, and use a bit of water to seal nori in place.
5. Let sit for a few minutes before cutting roll into 6 or 8 pieces.
6. Use tamari sauce (healthier than soy sauce) to dip your sushi.

Green Beans and Brown Rice in Curry Sauce

Serves 1 to 2

1/2 cup of brown rice, soaked

1 tbsp curry powder

6 carrots, juiced

1/2 small beet, juiced

1 stalk celery, juiced

2 tbsp ground flaxseeds

1 clove garlic, grated

1/2 small onion chopped finely

1 tbsp olive oil

Handful green beans, chopped

1. Soak brown rice in plenty water for 12 hours. Drain.
2. Mix in chopped green beans and place in serving dish.
3. In a glass, place onions, garlic and any other desired seasoning greens. Just cover these with olive oil and let soak.
4. In another glass mix curry powder with enough olive oil to make into a paste.
5. Juice beet, carrots and celery. Add curry (from step 4) and ground flaxseeds to juice and mix well. Pour curry sauce into serving sauce bowl.
6. Pour curry sauce over rice and green beans as desired. Add the seasoning mixture and enjoy!

Desserts

What's so wonderful about these desserts is that not only are they vegan and raw but they taste absolutely delicious! I would even recommend many of these desserts for athletes as a pre-game snack because of their high quality nutrients and simple fruit sugars. Although I do not recommend over consuming anything sweet (ie. these desserts), especially if you're not very active, they are not nearly as detrimental to your body as are conventional baked goods and traditional desserts. As with all the other recipes in this book, these desserts are "living" foods which means that they have their enzymes intact. The enzyme quality alone can turn a would-be sugary dessert into a nutritious snack that won't cause you to put on weight or feel like death! Remember, when foods contain their enzymes they don't get stored as fat in your body as readily as cooked foods.

Need proof? Look no further than my girlfriend's mother who has a natural sweet tooth. She might have one of these desserts each day. In fact, she probably eats more sweets than anyone I know! Amazingly, though, she has continued to maintain a very light body weight – she could actually stand to gain a few pounds. I guess that I should also mention that she previously lost about 30 lbs eating these desserts and many of the other raw dishes in this book!

So enjoy these desserts in moderation (especially if you have blood sugar issues) and don't feel guilty. Yes, they are dishes that are higher in sugar but they do contain quality ingredients and will provide great nutrition in comparison to baked/cooked desserts!

Chocolate Mousse

Serves 1 to 2

1 cup water

½ cup walnuts (unsoaked)

4 dates (pitted not soaked)

2 tbsp cacao powder

1 tsp vanilla extract

½ tsp cinnamon

¼ tsp nutmeg

1. Put 1 cup of water in your high speed blender (or food processor) then add enough walnuts to bring it up to 1 1/2 cups and blend until smooth.
2. Add the rest of the ingredients and blend until smooth

Sunset Pudding

Serves 2 to 3

2 bananas

1 mango, skinned and stoned

10 strawberries

2 tbsp ground flaxseed

2 dates, pitted and chopped (optional, because this is a very sweet pudding)

1. Put everything in a food processor and blend until it looks like a pudding.

Chocolate Energy Pudding

Serves 2 to 3

1 bananas
1/3 cup cacao powder
3-4 tbsp agave nectar
2 tbsp ground flaxseed
3-4 tbsp coconut oil (softened)
¼ cup water or coconut water

1. Put everything in a food processor or blender and blend until smooth.
2. May be stored in refrigerator but it will become more solid as the coconut oil hardens. Simply let stand in a warm room for 30 minutes before serving.

Banana Pudding

Serves 2

2 bananas
¼ cup dried coconut
2 tbsp raw agave or raw honey
1 tbsp coconut butter
½ lemon, juiced
1 tbsp lemon zest

1. Put everything in a food processor or blender and blend until smooth.

Raw Chocolate

Makes 6 to 8 (2" x 2" squares)

½ cup cacao nibs

½ cup cacao powder

¾ cup raw cashews

1 tbsp coconut butter

¼ cup agave

1 tsp vanilla

1. Put everything in a food processor and blend until thick.
2. Store in freezer

Orange Coconut Fudge

Makes 5 to 6 cups

5 cups dried shredded coconut

Juice of 1 orange

1 tbsp orange zest

½ cup agave nectar

1 tsp vanilla

1. Blend the coconut in a high speed blender until it becomes butter-like.
2. Add the agave, vanilla, and orange juice/zest and mix well.
3. Spoon contents onto a backing sheet and lay a sheet of plastic wrap over top.
4. Pat into a slab about ¼ inches thick and chill in the refrigerator before cutting (be careful to not over-chill the fudge or it will become too hard to cut).

Coconut Chocolate Truffles

Yields 36 truffles

2 cups dates, pitted

2 cups pecans, soaked 2 to 4 hours

1 tbsp cacao powder

1 tsp vanilla

½ cup dried shredded coconut

1. Throw all ingredients into a food processor and blend until the mixture becomes smooth and forms a ball.
2. Roll mixture into small balls (should yield about 36) and roll in shredded coconut for coating.

Pistachio Halvah

Serves 8

2 cups tahini (ground sesame seeds)

½ cup honey or agave nectar

1 tsp vanilla extract

½ cup pistachios, shelled (you can substitute with almonds if desired)

1. Process the tahini, honey, vanilla extract in a food processor.
2. Grind pistachios in a food processor, add to ingredients in step 1, and shape into a loaf.
3. Chill in the refrigerator for 2 hours. Slice into thick pieces and serve.

Banana and Strawberry Cream Pie

Serves 8

For the crust:
2 cups pecans
4 to 6 dates, pitted
1 tsp cinnamon

1. To make the crust, combine the pecans and dates in a blender. Combine well and then press into a pie dish. Sprinkle with cinnamon.

For the filling:
2 to 3 ripe bananas, sliced

2. Add sliced bananas on top of the crust.

For the topping:
¾ cup fresh strawberries
1 cup macadamia nuts or cashews, or 4 to 6 soaked dates

3. In a food processor, blend strawberries, nuts/dates, and just enough water to get the mixture moving.
4. Pour the mixture over the pie and decorate with whatever you like.
5. Refrigerate the pie to give it a more solid consistency.

Raspberry Cheesecake

Serves 8

For the crust:
2 cups macadamia nuts
4 to 6 dates, pitted
¼ cup dried shredded coconut

1. Sprinkle dried coconut onto the bottom of 8 or 9 inch springform pan.
2. In a food processor, combine nuts and dates. Press this mixture onto the coconut in the pan.

For the cheese:
3 cups cashews, soaked for at least 1 hour
¾ cup fresh squeezed lemon juice
¾ cup honey or agave nectar
¾ cup coconut oil
1 tbsp vanilla extract
Pinch of sea salt

3. In a food processor, blend all ingredients until smooth.
4. Pour this mixture onto the crust.
5. Place in the freezer until firm; remove cake from pan while frozen and place on a serving platter.

For the raspberry sauce:
2 cups raspberries
4 to 6 dates, pitted

6. Process raspberries and dates in a food processor until well blended and add on top of the rest of the cake.

Strawberry – Banana Gelato

This is a wonderfully delicious dessert on a hot summer's day. You can also use any of your other favourite berries instead of strawberries.

Serves 2

2 ripe bananas, frozen
2 cups strawberries, frozen

1. Peel and chop ripe bananas and store in freezer until frozen. Freeze strawberries as well.
2. Place frozen fruit in a food processor and blend until creamy smooth.

Smoothie &
juice GUIDE

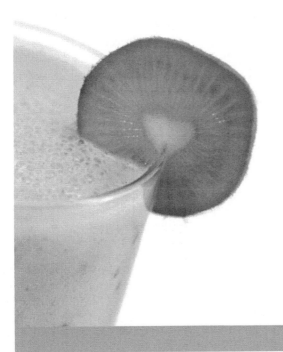

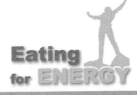
Eating for ENERGY

Smoothies

Smoothies are a great way of to get in tons of nutrients with little effort and minimal strain on your digestive system. They are well balanced between carbohydrates, amino acids (proteins), and healthy fats, and are highly recommended for those who don't have time or don't feel like preparing meals. There are also some great pre- and post-exercise smoothies that will help you recover better, become stronger, and develop greater endurance.

Many of these smoothies are also great for breakfast. Very often, I'll just have a smoothie in the morning and I'm good to go for a few hours. The wonderful thing is that you can be creative and add whatever ingredients you like and whip them up!

When preparing these smoothies, don't feel constrained. If you want to remove or add ingredients go right ahead. The goal is that you become comfortable enough to create your own smoothies. It's really pretty simple.

Choose a base such as water or nut milk, and add in some fruit or vegetables, and whichever boosting ingredients you like.

The **boosting ingredients** include:

- Whey/hemp protein
- Ground flaxseeds
- Spirulina
- Fish/flax/hemp oil
- Glutamine
- Sesame/Pumpkin seeds
- Coconut butter/oil

Meals don't have to be solid. As you will see in the following recipes, you can get plenty of high quality nutrition in liquid format – great on the go foods!

To help you construct your own smoothies, I've attached a vitamin and mineral chart so you can gain better understanding of vital nutrients and their sources.   Let this knowledge empower you to create your own great tasting concoctions!

Vitamins and Minerals

Health Benefits and Food Sources

VITAMIN	HEALTH BENEFITS	FOOD SOURCES
A	Antioxidant. Keeps skin and vision healthy. Anti-cancer.	Carrots, mangoes, melons, tomatoes.
E	Antioxidant. Good for blood cells, muscles, and nervous system. Protects against heart disease and cancer.	Fresh almond milk, sesame/pumpkin seeds.
K	Helps prevent osteoporosis. Ensures normal blood clotting.	Carrots, parsley, strawberries.
C	Antioxidant and anti-allergenic. Improves iron absorption and wound healing. Helps immunity and blood fat levels.	Citrus fruits, kiwis, guavas, mangoes, papayas, leafy greens, strawberries.
B1 (thiamin)	Aids metabolism. Maintains healthy nerves and muscles.	Carrots, oranges, nuts, avocado, seeds.
B2 (riboflavin)	Helps energy release from food. Keeps mucous membranes in good condition.	Fresh almond milk, cherries, cucumber, grapes, fish oil
B3 (niacin)	Helps maintain optimum energy levels. Keeps skin and mucous membranes in good condition.	Apples, apricots, bananas, lemons, pears, tomatoes, dates, figs.

B5 (pantothenate)	Anti-stress! Helps maintain energy levels. Aids antibody production. Protects against hypertension and allergy.	Honey, tomatoes, avocados.
B6 (pyridoxine)	Supports the nervous system. Aids hemoglobin production. May protect against PMS, asthma, migraine, and depression.	Bananas, oranges, tomatoes, fish oil, walnuts, spinach, avocados.
B7 (Biotin)	Maintains condition of skin, hair, sweat glands, nerves, and bone marrow. Aids fat metabolism and encourages appetite.	Fresh almond milk, bananas, red currants, carrots, leafy greens.
B9 (Folate)	Aids growth and development of a healthy nervous system.	Apples, beets, carrots, oranges, leafy greens, spinach.
B12 (Cobalamin)	Supports growth. Maintains health of the blood, bone marrow, and nervous system.	Fish oil, fermented soy, some sprouts.

MINERAL	HEALTH BENEFITS	FOOD SOURCES
Calcium	Gives structure and strength to bones and teeth. Maintains health of heart, nerve, and muscle tissues.	Sesame seeds, leafy greens, carrots, lemons
Sodium	Helps regulate fluid balance in the body.	Celery, beets, carrots, sea vegetables.
Copper	Maintains healthy red blood cells and bone and nervous tissue. May help protect against osteoporosis.	Beets, cherries, grapes, honey, melons, oranges, pineapples.
Sulfur	Enzyme reactions and protein building. Formation of collagen for healthy elastic skin.	Leafy greens, raspberries, radishes, sea vegetables.
Iodine	Supports growth, metabolism, and tissue repair.	Garlic, honey, lettuce, fish oil, sea vegetables.
Iron	Enables oxygen transport in the blood and muscles. Maintains energy. Supports nerves. Aids liver function.	Raspberries, strawberries, watermelon, apples, parsley, leafy greens.
Magnesium	Maintains bones and teeth. Protects against epilepsy, heart disease, hypertension, PMS, osteoporosis, mental illness. Relaxes.	Almond milk, leafy greens, apples, bananas, beets, oranges, cacao.

Manganese	Helps protein and fat metabolism. Keeps cell membranes healthy. May protect against diabetes, heart disease, epilepsy, cancer, and rheumatoid arthritis.	Bananas, blackberries, carrots, celery, ginger, oranges, pears, nuts.
Phosphorus	Supports the immune system and helps maintain energy. Important for bone health.	Carrots, parsley, raspberries.
Potassium	Regulates water balance and acid-base balance in the blood and tissues. Boosts energy and strength.	Bananas, leafy greens, tomatoes, nuts, seeds.
Selenium	Antioxidant. Enables red blood cells to function properly.	Celery, fish oil, Swiss chard.
Zinc	Aids wound healing. Maintains skin health. Protects against prostate disorders and mental disturbances. Helps regulate blood fat levels.	Beets, carrots, lettuce, oranges, peaches, tomatoes, pumpkin seeds.

Nut Milks

Since we've agreed that conventional pasteurized dairy is not our body's friend, the alternative lies in nut milks. Nut milks are exactly what they imply – non-dairy, antibiotic-free, liquid refreshment from ground nuts. They act as the base for many of the recipes in this book. Although almond milk is mainly emphasized in most of these recipes, feel free to use any other nuts or seeds you prefer. Nuts such as macadamia, cashew, and pecan are great and you can also use seeds like pumpkin, sesame, sunflower, and hemp to make milk.

I recommend using a high speed, high powered blender or Vita-mix when making nut milk. Conventional blenders will be less likely to finely grind the nuts/seeds. When making your nut milks in a conventional blender, it's best to start out with just enough water to cover the nuts/seeds and blend until combined. This will ensure the blades proper contact with the nuts/seeds. Once the initial nuts/seeds have been ground you can add more water. If small chunks are still present simply pour the milk through a cheese cloth or fine strainer.

When you have chosen your desired nut/seed milk be sure to soak the given nut/seed in filtered or spring water for at least 4 hours before-hand. Once they have been soaked, rinse them and then place them back in a fresh bowl of water in the refrigerator until you're ready to use them. Soaking nuts/seeds disengages their enzyme inhibitors and brings them back into an energetic and enzymatic living state. For this reason they should be kept in water in the refrigerator for a maximum of 3 days. I usually put a bunch of almonds in water before I go to bed so that they're ready to blend in the morning.

Almond Milk #1

Makes about 4 cups

1 cup raw almonds, soaked for 4 hours or more
4 cups filtered/spring water
¼ cup agave nectar or raw honey
Pinch of sea salt
A few drops of natural almond extract (optional)

1. In a powerful blender, blend the raw almonds and water at high speed for about 2 minutes.
2. If needed, strain the milk through a cheesecloth or fine strainer.
3. Rinse blender and then place almond milk with remaining ingredients back into blender and give it a whirl.

Almond Milk #2

Makes about 4 cups

1 cup raw almonds, soaked for 4 hours or more
¼ cup dates, pitted and soaked
4 cups of filtered/spring water
2 tbsp cinnamon
1 tbsp nutmeg

1. same procedure as in Almond Milk #1

Spinach Pear Smoothie

Serves 1 to 2

3 cups spinach

1 pear

¼ cup parsley

1 cup celery juice

Juice of half a lemon

1. Blend all ingredients into a blender until smooth.

Egg Nog #1

Serves 4 to 6

6 cups nut milk

1 cup soft dates

2-3 cups frozen bananas

2-3 tbsp of pumpkin pie spice

pinch of salt

1. Blend all ingredients in a blender until smooth

Egg Nog #2

Serves 1 to 2

1 cup water
1/3 cup soaked cashews
1 tsp nutritional yeast
¾ tsp vanilla extract
dash cinnamon
4 tsp agave
1 tsp coconut butter
pinch of sea salt

1. Blend all ingredients in a blender until smooth

Durian Smoothie

Serves 1 to 2

1 banana
1 mango
¼ durian fruit
vanilla, to taste
lemon juice, to taste

1. Blend all ingredients in a blender until smooth

Cinnamon Banana Smoothie

This smoothie tastes so good. I'll leave at that. Well ok maybe not. The bananas provide a great source of carbohydrates and electrolytes and the cinnamon acts to moderate their consequent effect on your blood sugar. Great for a pre- and post-workout snack.
Serves 1 to 2

2 bananas
1 ½ cups of almond milk
2 tbsp agave nectar
1 tsp vanilla extract
½ teaspoon ground cinnamon
pinch of sea salt
a few ice cubes (optional)

1. Blend all ingredients in a blender and enjoy!

Chocolate Banana Smoothie

Same as above but with raw cacao (chocolate) instead of cinnamon.
Serves 2 to 4

2 bananas
1.5 cups of almond milk
2 tbsp agave nectar
1 tsp vanilla extract
1 to 2 tbsp of organic cocoa powder
Pinch of sea salt
A few ice cubes (optional)

Thick 'n Creamy Chocolate Banana Milkshake

This is an awesome smoothie to make on a warm day. The trick is to cut up the bananas beforehand and store them in the freezer until they are frozen. When blended they replace the creaminess of ice cream.

Serves 2 to 4

2 bananas, chopped and frozen ahead of time

1 ½ cups of water or coconut water

2 tbsp agave nectar

1 tbsp of coconut butter/oil

1 tsp vanilla extract

1 to 2 tbsp of organic cocoa powder

Pinch of sea salt

4-5 ice cubes

1. Blend all ingredients except for the bananas and ice cubes.
2. Once mixture is consistent, add frozen bananas and ice cubes and blend until smooth and thick.

Blueberry Sunrise

A beautiful looking smoothie that is full of anti-oxidants (blueberries), natural digestive enzymes (pineapple), and wholesome goodness.

1 cup blueberries
2 cups pineapple, chunked
1 banana
1 cup diced mango
1 ½ almond milk or coconut water
3 tbsp agave nectar
2 tsp vanilla extract
pinch of sea salt

1. In a blender, puree blueberries with half of all ingredients. Pour this mixture into a glass.
2. Add remaining ingredients into blender and puree. Using the back of a spoon, gently pour this mixture overtop the existing "blue" mixture in the glass.
3. Have a look at your beautiful creation and then enjoy!

Monkey Mudslide

A filling drink that really hits the spot when you've got a craving for sweets yet it is moderated by the fiber and healthy fat of the flax seeds.
Serves 1 to 2

3 cups almond milk
2 bananas
4 dates, pitted and soaked (for at least 1 hour)
2 tbsp ground flax seed

1. In a blender, blend all ingredients until smooth.

Liquid Candy

Serves 1 to 2

1 mango

1 banana

½ cup strawberries

1 tbsp fish oil

1 tbsp ground flax seed

¼ cup walnuts, soaked

½ to 1 cup water, depending on thickness desired

1. Place all ingredients in a blender and give it whirl.

Nutty Banana

A close cousin to the Monkey Mudslide, this one provides more protein content and will keep you full for a little while longer.

Serves 1 to 2

1½ cups almond milk

1 banana

2 tbsp almond butter (raw if possible)

1 tbsp cacao powder

1 tbsp ground flax seed

½ tsp cinnamon

½ tsp nutmeg

5 ice cubes

1. Place all ingredients in a blender and blend until smooth.

Blood Oxygen Smoothie

This vitamin C, flavonoid, and iron-rich smoothie will give your blood a helping hand. The vitamin C in the orange helps the uptake of the iron in the pumpkin seeds.

Serves 1 to 2

1 banana

1 orange

2 cups cold water

2 tbsp pumpkin seeds

1 tbsp ground flax seed

1 tbsp hemp protein powder

1 tbsp agave nectar

1 tbsp hemp or flax oil

1. In a blender, blend all ingredients until smooth.

Enzyme Booster

Papayas and pineapples contain the enzymes papain and bromelain, respectively, which greatly assist in digestive function. They are also terrific for healthy skin as they are excellent sources of calcium, vitamin A, and vitamin C.

Serves 2 to 3

2 cups diced pineapple

2 cups diced papaya

1½ cups coconut water

2 tbsp agave nectar

2 tbsp vanilla extract

juice of ½ a lime

pinch of sea salt

1. In a blender, blend all ingredients until smooth.

Exercise Rejuvenator

This is one of my personal favourites for after a hard exercise session. It combines all the necessary post-exercise elements: simple sugars, healthy fats, easily assimilated amino acids, electrolytes, anti-oxidants, calcium, iron, and zinc.

Serves 1 to 2

2 cups almond milk (or coconut water)
1 banana
½ cup blueberries
1 tbsp ground flax seed
1 tbsp hemp protein powder
1 tbsp ground sesame seeds
1 tbsp pumpkin seeds
1 tbsp flax/hemp/fish oil
2-3 ice cubes (if desired)

Strawberry Smoothie

Serves 1 to 2

10 strawberries
1-2 tbsp coconut oil (softened)
1 tbsp agave nectar
1 tsp vanilla extract
Sprig of mint (optional garnish)

1. Blend all ingredients in a blender until smooth
2. Garnish with fresh mint

The Ironman

Red fruits, especially berries, contain high amounts of iron. Red watermelon has the highest iron content of any fruit and parsley has the highest iron content of any green-leafy vegetable. This is an amazing smoothie for anyone low in energy or anemic, and for women before, during, and after menstruation.

Serves 1 to 2

10 strawberries
10 raspberries
1 slice of watermelon
1 handful of parsley
½ cup of water
2-3 ice cubes (if desired)
a squeeze of lemon

1. In a blender, blend all ingredients until smooth.

Tropical Cocktail

Serves 1 to 2

½ guava, peeled and pitted
¼ pineapple, peeled
½ mango
2 lychess, peeled and pitted
1 tbsp ground flaxseed
Slice of lime (optional garnish)

1. Blend all ingredients in a blender until smooth
2. Garnish with slice of lime

Super Anti-Oxidant Smoothie

Berries are a terrific source of anti-oxidants and help build healthy blood. This "meal" is well balanced through the protein and trace minerals in the spirulina and the omega-3 fatty acids in the flax oil. The pectin and insoluble fiber of the apple and pear are also helpful in stimulating proper bowel function. One of these a day will keep disease away!

Serves 1 to 2

1 apple

1 pear

¼ cup blueberries

¼ cup raspberries

¼ cup blackberries

¼ cup strawberries

2 tbsp spirulina

2 tbsp flax oil

2 tbsp raw cacao powder (optional – cacao is the #1 source for anti-oxidants)

1. Blend all ingredients in a blender.
2. Add water until desired consistency is reached

Spinach Smoothie

Serves 1 to 2

2 cups fresh spinach

½ papaya, chopped

1 handful of parsley

1 handful of dandelion root

1 – 2 bananas

The freshly squeezed juice of 4 oranges

1. Throw all ingredients into a blender; blend until smooth

Banana Fig Smoothie

Serves 1 to 2

2 cups water

1 banana

4 fresh figs, hard stemmed removed

1 tbsp ground flaxseed

1 tbsp cinnamon

1. Throw all ingredients into a blender; blend until smooth

Grape and Fig Detoxer

Grapes are among the most cleansing fruit. Do your best to find organic and seeded grapes (the seeds are high in antioxidants). Grapes are also a terrific source of resveratrol, a compound known to thwart cancer growth and cardiovascular disease. Figs are one of the most potent mucus dissolving foods – great for those with a history of dairy!

Serves 2 to 4

4 cups red or green grapes (with seeds if possible)

1 cup fresh figs, hard stems removed

1 cup water

1 tbsp ground flaxseed

1 tsp vanilla extract

1 tbsp cinnamon

2 cups ice cubes

1. Throw all ingredients into a blender; blend until smooth

Green Monkey Smoothie

Serves 1 to 2

2 tbsp tahini (ground sesame seeds)

1 cup water

1 banana

½ cup chopped kale

½ cup chopped collards

½ cup chopped spinach

A handful parsley

2 tbsp dried (or fresh) mint

1 tbsp agave nectar

1. Blend all ingredients in a blender until smooth.

Aurora Borealis

Serves 1 to 2

½ cup raspberries

Juice of ½ lemon

1 tbsp agave nectar

½ nut milk of choice

1. Blend all ingredients together in a blender and serve.

Bananamania

Serves 1 to 2

1 banana
½ cup coconut meat (or solid coconut oil)
½ nut milk of choice
1 tbsp agave nectar

1. Blend all ingredients together in a blender and serve chilled.

Apricot Delight

Serves 1 to 2

4 fresh apricots, pitted
1 banana
½ nut milk of choice
1 tsp cinnamon

1. Blend all ingredients together in a blender and serve.

Sunrise Smoothie

Serves 1 to 2

1 banana

1 cup freshly squeezed O.J. (roughly 2-3 oranges)

1 cup strawberries

1 tbsp flax oil

1. Using a citrus juicer, juice oranges
2. All orange juice and all other ingredients into a blender and process until smooth.

Fresh Pressed Juices

If you're looking for an easy solution to consuming huge amounts of essential nutrients, this is it. Fresh juices combine tons of great ingredients destined to nourish, alkalize, and energize your body. I'll usually prepare a green juice after my morning run, which fuels me for several hours! They are pure energy! It's funny, since I've started eating predominantly whole living foods, I am amazed at how much of a liquid diet I have adopted. It must be because these juices (and smoothies) are easy to make, easy on the digestive process, chock-full of nutrients, and save me so much time. All you need to prepare them is a juicer.

Many of these juices are also great to enjoy on a warm summer's day. Just pour over ice, pull up a patio chair, and sip away!

Green Cappuccino

This is my morning power drink. I usually have it after my runs because it provides some simple sugars, great alkalinity, and an excellent source of amino acids (through the leafy greens). I call it "cappuccino" for the frothiness that tops off the juice.
Serves 1 to 2

8 stalks (leaves) of kale
4 stalks of celery
1 apple
½ cucumber
1 carrot
½ handful of parsley

1. Throw all ingredients into a juicer. Once juiced, give it a stir and enjoy!

Yerry and Yammy's Green Juice

I named this one after my girlfriend and mine's nicknames and because we tend to drink this when we just feel like an onslaught of pure alkalinity. This is a very detoxifying juice which can be used after a day of "not-so-good" eating.

Serves 1 to 2

4 stalks of kale
4 stalks of collard greens
2 leaves of swiss chard
1 handful of spinach
1 cucumber
2 stalks celery
1 pear

1. Place all ingredients through a juicer and drink promptly.

Blue-Green Orange Bliss

This is an easy to prepare concoction and is great 30-45 minutes before an exercise session as it provides great amounts of simple sugars that are well balanced by amino acids of the blue-green algae and the omega-3's of the flax seed oil – which means that your blood sugar is better maintained. Oh yeah, it also provides huge amounts of vitamin C and tremendous alkalinity.

Serves 1 to 2

5 oranges
1-2 tbsp of blue-green algae (ie. spirulina, chorella, etc...)
2 tbsp of flax oil

1. Juice of the oranges using a citrus juicer (or other tool)
2. Add blue-green algae to a glass and stir in orange juice and flax seed oil.

Athlete Booster

Spirulina is the highest protein food on the planet. Coconut water is the highest source of electrolytes found in nature. Both spirulina and coconut are alkaline and can help buffer lactic acid. Coconut oil also contains a unique group of healthy fatty acids known as MCTs (medium-chain triglycerides) that are quickly metabolized by the liver for quick energy!

Serves 1 to 2

2 cups coconut water
2 tbsp of spirulina

1. Combine both in a glass and stir

Sunrise Cocktail

Serves 1 to 2

1 oranges
1 tangerine
1 pink grapefruit
1 tbsp of flax/fish oil

1. Juice of the fruit using a citrus juicer (or other tool)
2. Add flax/fish oil and stir.
3. You can garnish with a segment of tangerine.

Apple-Pear Morning Pick Me Up!

Serves 1 to 2

4 apples
2 pears
Juice of ½ lemon
1 tbsp agave nectar

1. In a juicer, juice apples and pears.
2. Add the agave nectar and lemon juice, mix well, and enjoy!

Morning Glory

Serves 1 to 2

1 apple
1 large tomato
2 carrots
Juice of 1 orange
Slice of lemon (optional garnish)
Sprig of mint (optional garnish)

1. In a juicer, juice the apple, tomato, and carrots.
2. Add the orange juice, mix well, and enjoy!

Apple Spritzer

This is a wonderful drink on a hot summer's day. Plus, eating apples on a regular basis has been shown to improve breathing and lung function.

Serves 1 to 2

4 apples
Juice of ½ lemon
½ cup fizzy/sparkling water
2-3 ice cubes

1. In a juicer, juice the apples
2. Add the lemon juice and fizzy water and serve over ice!

Popeye's Secret

Serves 2

4 cups spinach, tightly packed
2 carrots, top removed
4 tomatoes
1 cucumber
Juice of ½ lemon

1. In a juicer, juice all ingredients and mix well.

Cabbage and Carrot Juice

This is a great juice for helping heal you gut and the mucosal lining of your digestive system.

Serves 1 to 2

1 head of cabbage
6 carrots, top removed
½ inch piece of ginger

1. In a juicer, juice all ingredients and serve immediately.

Grape-Celery Cooler

Serves 1 to 2

1 cup sweet red grapes
3-4 celery stalks
Mint for garnish (optional)

1. In a juicer, juice all ingredients and garnish with mint if desired.

Spicy Pear

Serves 1 to 2

4 pears
4 stalks celery carrots, top removed
1 tsp cinnamon

1. In a juicer, juice pears and celery.
2. Add cinnamon, stir well and serve.

Green Lemonade

Serves 1 to 2

5 apples
1 bunch of kale
4 stalks celery
1 grapefruit
Juice of 1 lemon

1. In a juicer, juice all ingredients, squeeze in lemon juice, mix well and serve.

Pineapple Fruit Cocktail

Serves 2

¼ **medium pineapple**

2 pears

1 inch fresh ginger

1. In a juicer, juice all ingredients, pour over ice, and serve.

The Friendly Thai

Serves 2

6 to 8 large leaves kale, collards, Swiss chard, or a combination.

1 small bunch cilantro

¼ **medium pineapple**

Juice of 2 limes

1. Run all ingredients through a juicer.
2. Squeeze in lime juice, stir, and enjoy.

Cucumber Summer Breeze

Cucumbers are hydrating, alkalizing, and cooling. They to help to flush wastes through the kidneys and dissolve uric acid accumulations commonly found in kidney and bladder stones. Celery also contains a lot of natural sodium to help keep you hydrated.

Serves 2

1 large cucumber
2 stalks celery
1 small handful fresh mint (plus additional for garnish)
Juice of 2 limes

1. Run all ingredients through a juicer
2. Squeeze in lime juice, stir, and pour over ice.
3. Garnish with mint sprigs if desired.

Skin Regenerator

This is drink is better than having a facial. Radishes and watercress are especially rich in sulfur, a mineral which helps builds collagen, a vital nutrient for skin elasticity. Grapes are full of essential fatty oils and antioxidants that protect your skin against free radical damage from the sun's UV rays.

Serves 2

½ cup chopped radish
1 large cucumber
½ bunch watercress (or 4 to 5 kale leaves)
4 cups green grapes
Small knob of fresh ginger

1. Run all ingredients through a juicer

DON'T FORGET TO...

Claim Your **FREE** *Eating for Energy*

Book Bonuses Today!

Go to...

www.totalwellnessconsulting.ca/book_bonuses.html

...for all the great bonuses that complement

this book.

About the Author

Yuri Elkaim, BPHE, CK, RHN
Owner & Founder, Total Wellness Consulting

 Yuri Elkaim graduated *summa cum laude* with a Bachelors of Physical Education and Health from the University of Toronto. He is a Certified Kinesiologist and considered by many as Canada's Top Fitness and Wellness Coach. He is a Registered Holistic Nutritionist and the current Head Coach of Strength & Conditioning and nutrition for the University of Toronto men's soccer program.

He has 8 years of Strength & Conditioning and nutrition experience working with such companies as the *Sports Clubs of Canada & Station 7 Reebok*, and has also worked as a clinical intern at the *Sports Injury and Rehabilitation Centre Inc.*, in Toronto.

He is currently the founder and owner of Total Wellness Consulting, a leading health, fitness and wellness company offering health-conscious individuals innovative programs and technologies to help them reach their goals of physical and mental well being. Total Wellness Consulting is currently Canada's leader in developing total body workouts for iPods/MP3 players. We help people lose weight, feel great, and improve their overall level of fitness.

Professional and Amateur Soccer Experience

Before founding his company, Yuri enjoyed playing professional soccer for 3 years. As one of the top goalkeepers in Canada, he played two years with the *Toronto Lynx* of the North American A-League (2000, 2001) and one year with *Lille OSC* of the French 1st division (2003 – reserves). His playing career was also marked by stints with *Bolton Wanderers FC*, *Norwich City FC*, and *Sao Paulo FC*.

During his collegiate years, Yuri was named a 2-time All-Canadian, OUA All-Star, and team MVP/captain with the University of Toronto Men's Soccer team before acting as the program's Head Strength & Conditioning Coach, helping the team capture OUA gold and silver medals, and 2nd, 4th and 5th place finishes at the National Championships.

Yuri wrote the first ever off-season program and conditioning manual (85 pages in length) for the University of Toronto Soccer Program. With his help, since 2002, the Varsity Blues have consistently fielded some of the fittest men's soccer teams ever seen at the University of Toronto, consistently ranking in the top 3 soccer programs in the country.

Fitness Industry Innovator

Yuri is the creator of Total Wellness Consulting's revolutionary **MP3 guided workouts**, the only progressive lineup of MP3 workouts in Canada. Featuring **Fitter U™**, the world's only 12-week MP3 body shaping system, and the **Treadmill Trainer™** MP3 running series, these one-of-a-kind "audio" workouts are the next best thing to actually working with Yuri himself!

His approach to health and fitness is all about balance, both physically and mentally, and achieving one's true potential. Through properly prescribed functional exercise and nutrition programs, as well as attention to the inner person, Yuri has helped thousands of individuals reach new heights and achieve a greater quality of life.

Yuri, the Presenter and Media Expert

Yuri is a highly sought-after public speaker, promoting healthy active living. He has given such motivating talks to such companies as *Bank of Montreal, BNI, the Sports Clubs of Canada, Advocis*, as well as *Queen's University* in Kingston, Ontario.

He has shared his wealth of knowledge and expertise by publishing articles in *Beyond Fitness* Magazine, *Impact Magazine*, and *Fitness Business Canada* Magazine. He and his MP3 guided workouts have been featured in several media including: *Maximum Fitness Magazine, CityTV, Perfect Fit, CP24, 24 Hours, Calgary Herald, eTalk Daily*, and *Breakfast Television*.

If you would like to book Yuri for a speaking engagement or other media endeavour please call 416-885-9874 or send an email request to info@totalwellnessconsulting.ca

Become an Eating for Energy Affiliate and Earn Cash!!!

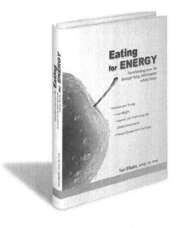

Have you enjoyed this book?

Would you recommend it to other people you know?

If so, why not get paid for each person you refer who buys Eating for Energy?!

All you have to do is logon to our website and click on the "Become an Affiliate" link and you will instantly earn a **50% commission** on any sales that result from your referrals. You will be supported with marketing materials and email scripts that you can send to your network immediately. Visit **www.totalwellnessconsulting.ca** to get started today!

Other Programs by Yuri Elkaim

These iPod/MP3 guided workout programs are available at the following sites:

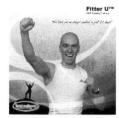

Fitter U™

www.myFitterU.com

12-week weight loss exercise program

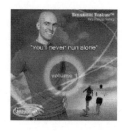

Treadmill Trainer™

www.myTreadmillTrainer.com

Running-specific cardio workouts

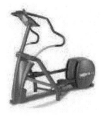

Elliptical Workouts

www.EllipticalWorkouts.com

Elliptical-specific cardio workouts

1722183R0021

Printed in Great Britain
by Amazon.co.uk, Ltd.,
Marston Gate.